Accidents Will Happen

By Martyn Quinlan

First Kindle edition 2013

For my wife

Preface

The year is nineteen ninety-two and Will is still a relatively young man but now he has to try to digress to the childhood that was snatched from him by the death of his brother to stop his near idyllic life from disintegrating.

Why has he begun to unravel now? It couldn't just be the death of his mother surely? Why so paranoid about the future existence of his native London or perhaps even the whole world even before the atrocities of 9/11 were ever conceived?

His new bride just wishes he would start to communicate. In logistical terms at least that could be so much harder before the introduction of mobile phones into everyone's life. You just have to look at the unfortunate James, the sad middle-aged man, who spends so much of his time and coins in filthy telephone boxes negotiating with his estranged wife.

What part does he have to play in this story? What is the point of James? He'd probably ask you that himself.

There you have it in essence, two men struggling to cope with the consequences that life's accidents have thrown at them. One accident that left broken bones and broken hearts and the other more profound and self-inflicted that took a good deal of hindsight and reflection to realise it had happened at all. Can either man recover and move on?

Foreword

All that remained from the fair were the plastic food wrappers and associated litter that had been blown into the thicker foliage of the surrounding woods so escaping the council sweep. A solitary balloon, having left its crying owner, sat deflated among the higher branches of a sycamore tree.

Matt got off the bus pulling clumsily at the bamboo stick until the little red net at its end became unfastened from the handrail by the door. Now he waited anxiously for his younger brother to come down from the seats at the back where he'd insisted on sitting.

'Come on Billy or it'll go!' He called angrily.

Billy finally stepped down into the blazing sunshine in his red shorts and the mustard tee-shirt which matched his oily hair. The unkempt locks ruffled by a warm brisk breeze. The boys walked the short distance to the zebra crossing indifferent to the panoramic views of London and far beyond. Billy held his big brother's hand without any prompting finding the speed and sheer volume of traffic breath-taking.

The nearest car stopped suddenly with a jolt, forcing those around it to an equally abrupt halt. An instantaneous chorus of horns echoed around the plateau growing louder as the traffic snarled its way back to the roundabout and around again to where the boys crossed, trapping itself then uncoiling impatiently as the youngsters mounted the pavement.

The sun dazzled them both in the reflection of the rippling pond as they approached it. They could barely contain their excitement now but there was still one more narrow road to negotiate and Matt pulled his brother back instinctively while they waited for a lull in the traffic before racing to the other side.

Once across Matt dropped the rod with a clatter against the large paving slabs and ran towards the water then, suddenly mindful that Billy may follow his lead and drop the glass jam jar he'd been carrying since home, turned to his brother and inspected both stubby empty hands.

'Where did you put the jam jar Billy?' He asked, but he didn't need a reply when he saw the horror on his brothers' face.

'You left it on the bus didn't you?'

'I jammed it between the chair and the window so that it wouldn't fall down.' Billy whimpered

'And you forgot it didn't you!' Matt roared as he rushed forward shoving Billy to the ground.

'I'm telling mum!' Billy screamed pushing himself up and away from his brother in one swift movement.

Matt clenched his teeth with rage but he knew the compulsion to be violent had already passed and now he watched his little brother from a distance picking away the dirt and tiny stones from the elbow he'd landed on and he was already sorry he'd pushed him.

'Let's look for the fish!' He called presently.

'But how we going to get them home now?' Billy asked gloomily.

'I'll go over to that pub!' Matt shouted as he pointed to the large white building just in view from where he was standing. Billy couldn't see it so hesitantly made his way back to his brother.

'Come on, I'm not going to get you.' Matt assured him.

'I'm still telling mum.' Billy warned clutching the bad elbow as he approached.

Billy faced where his brother was still pointing.

'Is it that white building there?' He asked.

'Yeah,' Matt confirmed 'that's Jack Straws' Castle... can you see the black writing?'

'Oh yeah!' Billy exclaimed excitedly 'But I can't read what it says!'

'It says 'Jack Straws' Castle,' Matt affirmed, 'and that's a pub.'

'Will they give you a jam jar then?' Billy enquired.

'Course they won't you idiot, but there's a garden round the side and everyone will be drinking outside today as it's so boiling and I'll go and get an empty beer glass from one of the tables when no ones' looking.'

'How'd you know there's a garden round the side?' Billy enquired.

'Cos mum and dad used to take us there when we were little.'

Billy pondered this for a moment then wondered why his brother was walking around the pond away from the pub until Matt explained that he wanted to make sure the fish were really in there before he took a chance to get the glass. Billy was upset that Matt still didn't totally believe him about the fish even though he'd sworn on their mum's life and he'd never say that if it wasn't true. Matt would have seen the lady and the man put the fish in himself if he hadn't been gawking up at the people on the big wheel when they were driving past and dad would have seen them as well if he hadn't been too busy driving.

'You go round the other way Billy,' Matt instructed, 'I'll meet you at the end...
and just remember,' he advised pointing at both of his eyes as he said it, 'keep 'em peeled.'

Billy smiled weakly then turned and walked in the direction his brother had requested him to.

The pond was almost triangular in shape and it was easily the most massive one Billy had ever seen. Matt looked titchy on the other side of it and it was a shame he was so far away because Billy wanted to know why it was called 'White Stone Pond' when there were red bricks all around it. He eventually resolved that the grey stuff at the bottom was just dirt which must've covered some white stones underneath it.

'I've found one!' Matt suddenly exclaimed.
Billy ran at an instant to get to his brother's position but Matt had called for him to stop and was jabbing his finger excitedly to somewhere in the middle of the water.

'There it is Billy... can you see it?' Matt asked, but Billy had become unsighted by the sun's fierce reflection which had sent a sharp pain through his eyes.

'Look Billy!' Matt persisted 'It's swimming towards you now!'
Billy tried following the path of his brother's pointed finger by using the palm of his hand as a shield against the light yet all he could see was the grey bottom and a few dunes of silt.

'There, Billy, there!' Matt cried and now Billy had seen a fish swim right up to the edge of the pond.

'I can see it!' He screeched.

'No not there, Billy, there!' Matt shrieked, specifying an area further within the pond.

'No, it's here, look!' Billy insisted pointing directly below him at the small fish.

'Wow!' Matt yelled deliriously, 'we've found both of them already!'

Billy raced around the edge toward his brother.

'Quick gimme the net!' He demanded as he ran.

Matt, becoming aware that the rod was still over on the paving stones, made a careful dash himself to ensure he reached it first.

'Let me have it!' Billy pleaded when he had reached his brother but Matt held the length of bamboo above his head and out of reach from Billy's clawing hands.

'Give it to me!' Billy shouted forcefully.

'No way!' Matt replied.

'Give it me! I saw him first!'

'So? It's my fishing net.' Matt reminded him.

'No it's not!' Billy contended, though he knew it was true and the leaps he was making to reach the rod high above his brother's head began to decrease in height once he'd realised he was never going to win the dispute.

Both boys went back to where Billy's fish had been but now it had gone and there was more disagreement as to which of their fault it had been to allow it to escape, then Matt reasoned that even if they had caught a fish they had nothing to put it in until they had got a beer glass.

Billy was left to guard their uncaught property while Matt gingerly made his way back over the narrow strip of road and onto the pavement that stretched around the bend to the pub. Matt had left the rod in his brothers charge and Billy was almost certain it would be his only chance all afternoon to catch a fish himself so he walked around the pond staring intently at the tiny waves that flicked against its boundaries hoping to be lucky enough to detect a flash of gold by the water's edge before Matt returned. He'd circled the pond half a dozen times before Matt came back without spotting either fish and although there was a decent breeze as there always was this high up, he'd become hot and exhausted by the

onerous heat of the sun and now his throat was dry and hot and he
wanted to drink something before, he imagined, he'd die of thirst.
He hadn't even noticed that his brother had reappeared empty
handed save for the crumpled plastic bag which he held firmly
through the cut-out handles while the rest of it flapped violently in
all directions at the slightest shift in wind.

'Couldn't find any glasses.' Matt stated cheerfully.
There hadn't been anyone drinking outside when he searched the
beer garden and there wasn't any litter or empty glasses or bottles
either. Still, Matt thought, it didn't matter because he'd found the
bag up against a fence and that was going to be a million times
better than any old glass or jam jar.

Billy squinted hard in concentration as he tried to understand
Matt's mood.

'Are we going home?' He asked.

'Course not.'

'Where are we gonna put the fishes now then?'
Matt held up the bag that had wrapped itself around his bony
elbow.

Billy screwed up his face again in confusion. Matt pulled the end
of the bag from his arm and held it out like a flag.

'And how's that s'pose to work?'

'Errr,' Matt began sarcastically 'how do you think they got here!'
saying each word slowly and deliberately as if explaining to
someone who was backwards.

Billy omitted a shrill burst of laughter as the penny dropped and
responded by pressing his tongue out from behind the skin under his
lower lip and grunting comically.

'Spaz!' Matt quipped and both boys chuckled as Billy held out the
rod for Matt to take.

They began their search of the pond again in the full blaze of the
yellow orb high above them. Matt stuffed the plastic bag into his
jeans and was stalking carefully around the perimeter with both
hands grasping the rod. Billy followed close behind and couldn't be
persuaded to start on the opposite side because there was stuff Billy
wanted to know so it was best he stayed with his brother so he

could ask things. First and the most important was when would Matt be going to buy some drink as Billy was gasping now. He'd offered to go himself but when he looked around there were still just as many cars racing each other and cutting one another up with the drivers bibbing their horns like it was always the other cars fault. It was so annoying Matt wouldn't go yet, even though he was thirsty too but he said they'd already wasted a lot of time.

Another question Billy wanted answered as they begun a second circuit was why had that lady and man put the fish in the water in the first place? If they didn't want goldfish why had they tried to win them?

'They probably forgot they didn't have a goldfish bowl.' Matt reasoned.

****

But reason or logic hadn't played any part in the actions of the two young lovers on the evening they had crouched down together with the setting sun rippling in golden threads across the pond and the pink clouds in the distance pointing towards tomorrow, both releasing the solemn little creatures from the meagre transparent cells that had borne them there into the dark inscrutable expanse of water. Perhaps there had been some rational thought behind it or was it just the sudden urge to demonstrate their new found sense of freedom? That giddy feeling experienced in the first throws of love.

****

'How can they live in there without food?' Billy enquired as the two boys continued their search.

'They probably eat flies and that.' Matt deliberated.

'But how many flies do you reckon fall in the water?' Billy wondered.

'I don't know!' Matt replied impatiently. 'They've only got tiny guts so just one fly would probably fill them up for a week!'

Content with the answer Billy closed his sticky mouth and drew the air through flared nostrils contemplating whether it had been long enough to bring up the question of them getting a drink again when Matt held his hand out to stop him in his tracks.

'Look.' Matt whispered pointing just below them.

The water lapped softly against the brick borders and the fish floated motionless except for the occasional steadying flap of a tiny fin. Matt licked his lips in anticipation like a hungry cat and lowered the net steadily into the water slowly enough not to break the surface into ripples but rather let it be hugged by the gentlest swell as it became submerged. Then there was a sudden plop as the lip went in and became engulfed by the waiting tide at its edges. The fish darted forward followed in a moment by a reckless jerk upwards from the net as Matt flicked both wrists hard against the bamboo rod. A few seconds past in confusion as the water which had clouded in the struggle began to settle and clear. The fish hadn't quite been caught but was trapped between net and brick. Matt having realised in time stopped pulling and held the rod calmly in position.

'Billy!' He screamed but his little brother was already crouching with his hand in the water at the base of the net and the fingers of his other hand were gently lifting the wide end upwards against the pond wall until the fish came tumbling from pond to brick and finally to the floor of the net where it writhed helplessly in the suffocating air.

'Where's the bag!' Matt barked anxiously.

'You've got it!'

Matt looked down and saw the mound of blue plastic protruding from his pocket then a small wet hand snatch at it. Billy waved the bag apart and thrust it awkwardly into the cool water. It hadn't stayed open but the water gradually seeped in until there was enough to fill the bottom and Billy pulled it out by its handles ignoring the cascade of water that had clung to the outside and made its way home via his legs and plimsolls. Now the handles were pulled open and the net gently placed within then tipped downwards . The boys watched the fish splash back into its own atmosphere then flit back and forth searching for an escape before slowing with the quick acceptance of its situation. The boys were overjoyed and grinned jubilantly at one another. Matt with the adult teeth he had yet to grow into and Billy with the gap where the adult teeth were yet to grow.

'Are we still going to call them Abbot and Costello?' Billy asked.
'Course.'

'Shall we wait and see which ones the fattest and which ones the thinnest before we call them their names.' Billy suggested.
'S'pose so.' Matt agreed.

Billy was pleased. Although he liked watching those old films with his brother he didn't like them enough to name the goldfish after them and anyway the fat one was really stupid and funny but the thin one was really miserable and boring. Billy hoped that neither fish was fat so they wouldn't know which one to call Abbot and which one Costello and then they'd have to call them something else. Matt took the bag from his brother and hooked it over an arm of one of the iron benches near where the pond was widest.

'Can we go and get a drink now?' Billy pleaded.
'Not now,' Matt answered sternly, 'we might as well wait until we've caught the other one then we can walk down the hill to the shop and then go to the bus stop down there.'

'But I'm dying of thirst!' objected Billy.
'So am I.' said Matt.

'Let's go and get a drink then you idiot!'
'No... I've already told you.' Matt muttered dismissively walking back to the pond and beginning his next journey around.

Billy was indignant. The heat beat down relentlessly and the whole area was awash in harsh sunlight. He could feel his arms burn and the sweat trickling down from his hair and armpits. His thirst had made his tongue cleave to the roof of his mouth. He'd decided. If Matt wouldn't get a drink he would.

When Matt had made a circuit, Billy was waiting for him by the bench.
'Give me some money, I'm gonna go myself.' He declared.

Matt continued to walk, eyes down, absorbed in his search.
'Give me some money!' Billy ordered as he followed his brother.
Matt still didn't look up but this time he answered.

'You can't cross the roads on your own.'
'There aren't even any roads going down the hill!'
   'Course there are!'
'No there's not!' Billy maintained, but he didn't really know and his ignorance and frustration made him erupt. The tears that suddenly came stung his eyes and blinded him as he ripped and clawed for the money in his brother's pockets.

   Matt held his balance and tried to swing his brother away with his hips but without success. Billy couldn't force his way into the pocket but he had caught Matt unexpectedly on the cheek with a fingernail as he flailed his arms in frenzy.

   Matt felt the sting of pain as the skin ripped and he let the rod fall releasing his arms to unleash his own fury. The blows fell heavily onto Billy's head. His brother's knuckles had always felt like steel. The fists gave a sharp intense pain then a dull numbness. Billy had got away but he was wailing behind the last bench in the agony of another defeat.

   Matt was worried now. He worried that Billy might have a bruise on his face or a lump on his head and his mum would kill him even when he explained it was self-defence and showed her the cut to prove it. Matt looked at the slow line of traffic directly across the pond. All those grown-ups alone in their cars with their windows wound down, looking. One could easily be a Cop. Better carry on he thought. Act normal. Billy was still crying into the crease of his arm and although Matt felt sorry, he knew he deserved it. He picked up the rod and went back to his job. He walked anti-clockwise now, away from Billy. He wanted everything to calm down again. He thought he'd seen something straight away but it was only a leaf. Two more trips around followed and he could see Billy had sat down on the bench where their fish was. He wasn't crying anymore, he just looked like he was sulking. That's when Matt had the next sighting. Billy saw his brother's animated frame get on tip toe with the rod held at full stretch above his head like an axe ready to fall. He didn't move for quite a while. The fish moved further down the pond but came closer in. Matt began to track it walking silently in almost slow motion as the fish came closer still.

13

Suddenly a shower of droplets appeared before him and from the corner of his eye he could see Billy running away having dispensed a hand full of gravel.

'Get lost!' he screamed venomously at the sneering figure of his brother as he ran away.

Turning back he scoured the target area but the fish had vanished.

The sun had visibly moved by the time Matt had seen that slight streak of gold again. It was too far away but it seemed to be working its way inwards towards the thin end of the pond where the driveway sloped into the water. Closer it came then out a little then closer still. Matt stood perfectly still with the rod poised. From close behind he heard his little brother's plimsolled footsteps smack against the paving stone then he saw him squat by the edge and scoop water up and out from the palms of his hands in the direction Matt was concentrating on.

'I'll kill yah!' Matt warned, holding his position where he could still see the fish, though he was tempted to throw down the rod again and chase the little div.

The fish seemed unaffected and drifted in the faint swell of current that hadn't as yet brought it near enough.

Billy resumed his spoiling trick from the other side but was too far away to do harm. After a time he drew nearer, unsure of the effect he was having on either fisher or fish. He scooped up the water again but still without consequence.

Matt, expressionless, watched from the corner of his eye as Billy grew bolder with each failed attempt. Matt sensed he was going to catch something soon.

Finally, Billy's effort was close enough and the startled fish sprang to its side and distanced itself from the disturbed water only to flip around just as swiftly bringing itself back from where it had fled. If anything, it had come closer to the reach of the net.

Matt couldn't bear to let Billy ruin things now and tried to reason with him.

'Don't muck about anymore,' he said genially 'and I promise I'll buy some drink.'

'What's that?' Billy teased.

'Don't muck about...' Matt began but Billy had already interrupted.

'Can't you talk any louder?' he taunted, 'don't you want me to make a noise?'

'Shut up or you're dead.' Matt threatened quietly.

Billy backed away but raised his voice higher still.

'What's the matter Mathew; don't you want me to scare the fish away?' He questioned loudly.

He could see Matt's face tighten and decided to sing to keep up the disturbance and slipped heedlessly into the whole act.

'I'll... be... your... long haired lover from Liverpool and I'll do anything you ask!' He sung with a grin like little Jimmy Osmond, legs kicking, arms flailing.

'You look like a right poof!' Matt spat at his brother to show his full disgust.

'Well, you love Jeremy Thorpe!' Billy retorted.

Matt turned back to the pond determined to ignore his tormentor as Billy started the routine again.

It wasn't so much what he was doing, but more how much he was enjoying it that finally cracked Matt's composure. Billy had begun another full tilted kick to coincide with the chorus of the song when it first registered that his brother had sprung towards him and in his panic he tried to recoil his foot to make his escape but in doing so had let his second foot chase the first, so that in one movement he had managed to launch both feet knee high into the air before him, forcing his shoulders to pitch backwards until the whole of his being was suspended momentarily in mid-air.

Matt stopped running and watched anxiously as his little brother descended onto the paving slabs, the coccyx of his spine taking the full brunt of impact. Leaping with fright he rushed to his brother's side. Billy sat legs splayed apart his eyes screwed shut and his mouth wide open as if to scream but all sound was lost as he struggled to cope with his breathlessness. Dirty tears trickled down his cheeks.

Matt had put his arm around his brother's back to comfort him and was frantically seeking assurance that he was okay with a bombardment of concerned questions.

Finally, Billy exhaled his discomfort with a deep groan then he was laughing as he cried and swivelling his hips as if to disperse the pain. As he regained his breathing he laughed even louder. Matt joined in, at first with relief then having had time to reflect on the accident he became resoundingly gleeful.

Both boys agreed it had been something just like you'd see in an Abbott and Costello film. They both took pleasure in re-enacting the experience several times over in slow motion refining their movements to exaggerate the comedy.

When their amusement had eventually abated Billy's thirst came back to the fore.

There was no question of Matt refusing him drink now.

They walked down the hill side by side, Matt swinging the rod and Billy careful not to swing the bag containing the fish.

They shared a large bottle of cream soda, drinking it outside the shop until it was empty and they could retrieve the deposit on the bottle. There was now just enough money for another bottle or a Fab ice lolly each.

They ate the lollies as they climbed back up the hill with the breeze cooling their faces and whisking the lolly wrappers back down the road. They were refreshed, quiet and thoughtful, their long shadows ahead of them. Billy wondered why the water inside the bag was so murky, as it had seemed so clear in the pond. Dirt clung to its insides and he worried that the fish would become ill.

Matt checked the bus fare again for fear of being stranded so far from home.

On their return they worked their way silently around the pond, Billy searching as diligently as his brother. There were sightings but always at a distance and as the sun sank lower the water turned gold obscuring their view. They searched until they were thirsty again, tired and disheartened. Billy had wanted to go sooner but Matt had been reluctant until a bus appeared at the brow of the hill ensnared in the rush hour traffic.

On the way home they promised each other they would return another day.

****

Billy sat on the back seat of the bus like before but now there was no one there to hurry him along but himself and as he rushed forward some of the water tipped from the plastic bag he was carrying and stained a leg of his jeans and splashed up at his shoes as it hit the rubber flooring.

When he clambered off, he was suddenly reminded of how cold it was. The wind threatened to hurl him and the bag in opposite directions so he clasped it carefully against his stomach then unzipped his parker coat far enough to slip the bag inside. Cold water seeped through his jumper making him shiver.

The traffic moved freer than the last time he was there but he still had to wait patiently at the zebra crossing until his presence was acknowledged by the slowing movement of cars and impatient stares from their drivers. He walked across awkwardly, hunched forward trying not to spill anymore, conscious of how silly he looked.

The second road proved more of an obstacle and although the flow of vehicles was more sporadic, he was too nervous to chance a slow crossing with the bag where it was and so took it out getting ever wetter as he did so.

The wind blew stronger and small waves tossed against the pond's wall spraying tiny droplets all over him.

He walked around the water's edge desperate to find the fish still there.

Billy's eyes watered and his nose ran uncontrollably as he was hit by a sharp cross wind. He wiped his nose with his sleeve, his eyes still intent on the task.

He'd lapped the pond countless times without seeing anything. The sun was already sinking behind the black and leafless trees and he was in the grip of persuading himself that his tears were all from the weather when something bright caught his eye just below his feet and almost knowingly the fish made its escape to the further reaches of its home.

Billy didn't think he'd miss Matt too much when he was gone. He had the bedroom to himself now and although Matt's bed was still there, he could use it as a mountain when he was playing with his soldiers. He played with the soldiers a lot and with his action men and he could use the whole edge of the bedroom to race his toy cars around.

When he couldn't think of anything else to do and he was really bored he really wished Matt was there to make up a game. Sometimes he would get an ache in his chest and it made him feel better to lie down on Matt's bed but this wasn't allowed anymore as the bed always needed to be remade. Instead Billy would kneel by its side and rest his head on the soft clean blanket with the palms of his hands laid flat and there he would stay with his eyes closed until he felt better.

One day as his mum entered the room to put away some shirts she had ironed she found him kneeling, eyes closed and she asked him if he was tired. Billy told her he wasn't.

It was that same day that he thought about Costello swimming around and around in his bowl and he wondered if he sometimes got an ache too. He was sure no one had even wondered if Costello was tired before.

Billy held the plastic bag by two corners, top and bottom, then tipped the water gently into the pond. In a moment he saw Costello splash into view and just as quickly swim away.

Billy patted his pockets and felt the jingle of coins for the bus. He waited for a gap in the traffic then raced across the narrow road.

James was bored and now to make matters worse the hand he had propped his head against had gone completely numb. He sat up and flapped the lower arm to bring back its circulation.

Simultaneously somewhere in the depths of the Amazon Rainforest, a beautiful Heliconius Sara butterfly began its descent to the safety of a dense clump of Heliconia flowers when a mysterious breeze swept it upwards again. At that moment an opportunist Humming bird seized the chance to swoop trapping the butterfly inside its hungry beak.

James yawned, a deep animated yawn to express his general disinterest to the empty room. Shall I make another mug of tea he pondered? Shall I just drown myself in bloody tea?

The diversions from the endless cackle of daytime television were slight in this room.

The splash stained kettle was perched in the corner on its wooden stand. The PG Tips in its box. The ragged bag of sugar and a milk carton that was always tepid given there was neither a fridge nor room for one. It wasn't a problem as long as James remembered to pour it away in the bathroom before it began to turn.

Other than that, there were the glass-fronted wardrobes' which, by their craft, made the space seem deceptively small rather than tiny. Then of course there was the single bed resting against the opposing wall. The bed he slept in and sat on and used as his dining table. There was nothing else but the badly tuned television set which only showed children's programmes at that time of day and the only other two activities he could think of that morning didn't take very long to perform.

He could either watch himself become sore with a further bout of self-abuse in the wardrobes reflection or he could make another mug of tea.

James reached over to the wooden stand and flicked the kettle back to life.

Not to worry he decided, not too long and *the Ricki Lake Show* would be on which he quite enjoyed. There was some primeval pleasure to be had watching this Lake woman trying to mediate between hapless fat women with three teeth and their cheating partners with none. That would pass the time.

James yawned once more and squeezed both functional fists tight to suppress that rancorous feeling he was trying so hard to ignore.

The holidays were the worst time of all. Why did he even bother having them when he couldn't see the kids? Why on earth was Debbie being so bloody-minded over custody anyway after all she'd done to him?

Other than the allotted weekends each fortnight when he was allowed to see the boys and even have them stay with him if he had somewhere to put them, he was only given a set two week access period for holidays which meant he had an additional thirteen days leave to contend with. God knows what he'd do with all the extra time off once his teaching job came through.

Steam rose from the boiling kettle as it switched itself off and James pushed himself up to stand in the narrow corridor between wardrobes and bed to make his drink.

He heard the music bring the present programme to an end. It was later than he thought so if he waited briefly the Lake woman would pop up with her show's preliminary slot.

He added the latest squeezed teabag to the mound that had risen on the stand waiting to be flushed down the loo and suddenly there she was.

'Today's topic!' the host announced passionately, 'Why... can't... I... see my Grandchild?'

She always seemed to do that sort of dramatic build up and under normal circumstances he would have welcomed the variation on the show's usual theme, but for now the subject was just a little too close to home for James to contend with.

He would have to find something else to watch on the other three channels.

Of course, he could always go out if he wanted to. One plus point about separation was the ability to please oneself.

He could always jump on a bus to Romford and visit *Parvs* Bar which he now considered himself to be a regular patron of, although he hadn't as yet become familiar enough to have a proper conversation with the other regulars. It was always going to be difficult with the music going at such a volume.

Still it was certainly an interesting venue with its white washed walls, pink alcoves and illuminates everywhere and what actually made the place fascinating were the two completely contrasting elements from which the clientele were based.

There was the trendy young crowd of girls and boys looking very much like they belonged and there was the older, balding collection of single men who probably didn't belong anywhere anymore. James, although in his early fifties, preferred to think of himself as a neutral observer rather than bracket himself into the latter group.

He found himself wondering what the bar would look like in daylight. Probably more bizarre than usual with most of the crowd at work and just the elderly custom scattered around the zinc topped tables enjoying the Stella Artois at only one pound a pint.

The prices to be honest were the only reason he and anyone over the age of twenty-one drank there. For all its faults, James quipped to his reflection, the place was reassuringly inexpensive.

It would be interesting to see whether the television screens that somehow hung from the ceiling by a whisker of metallic thread would still be blasting out the obscure hits from the MTV channel in the middle of the afternoon.

James pictured the screens flitting seamlessly from black boys jiggling their jewellery to black girls jiggling everything out of their bikinis.

Sometimes on the odd payday evening he would loiter longer than usual at the bar while his head swum with his favourite poison and he'd watch the kids actually make something of the music through dance. But then, he reflected, the inevitable drunken disputes would begin and the doormen would find themselves between opposing fists, chairs, ash-trays and once even bottles and a glass.

The toilets at *Parvs* suddenly appeared in his mind's eye. He couldn't help but marvel at the state they would get in as the night progressed. How did these kids get them like that in such a short space of time? Vomit, shit, piss all over the floor, an odd used condom floating contentedly in the solitary cubicle, the occasional splattering of blood across the grimy tiles.

They even made the loos in this awful place he lived in seem sanitary by comparison and drat, he'd probably need to go now that he'd thought of it. Emptying your bladder here was still a very unpleasant experience. At least at *Parvs* you were usually pie eyed enough not to care about the whole hygiene thing but here there were just two lavatories between nine rooms which he'd guesstimated at the last count meant seventeen people.

It wasn't so much that he seemed the only one willing to use the toilet brush when necessary, it was more about how the men were always splashing the seats.

Naturally both men and especially young boys couldn't help but miss the bowl every now and then from a standing position so why didn't they have more consideration for everyone else and sit down while they went? Surely their women must have complained?

In retrospect James didn't know if these women were the type to complain. These Bosnians or Kosovars or whatever they were. He'd never heard many raised voices from the other rooms in all the time he'd been there, certainly not from the women.

Still being oppressed by their men folk he presumed.

Having completed the tea making he made a quick jaunt down the corridor to the toilets before he had the time to change his mind.

He heard a muffled fart from the alcoholic Scotsman as he passed his room and wondered when on earth he ever did this site work he'd been talking about as James couldn't remember a time he'd ever known him to be out of the house.

Perhaps he'd got it wrong and had understood him less than he thought he had which seemed unlikely considering some of the other inmates who'd been learning English for less than a month or two were by his ear already more eloquent.

Still at least the Scotsman had inadvertently taught him an early lesson of not drinking alone in your room.

It would of course be a lot cheaper than even *Parvs* excellent value and he could chase away those despairing thoughts that seemed to creep up on him every so often in the dead of night, but where would it stop? Could it stop? James wasn't confident enough of his already strained self-control to find out and the way the Jock fellow shook was reason enough not to risk it.

Best leave things the way they are, he reiterated, rising from the toilet seat and dabbing his end dry with the single sheet of toilet paper he'd brought along. You couldn't leave a roll in there. Next time you went in it would all be gone and James couldn't afford it.

He was still in awe at how much that side of life had changed since the separation. He'd known roughly how much the mortgage repayments were and the cost of a year's road tax for the car, but other than that he was almost completely in the dark. His wife used to deal with all of that side of things: the household bills etcetera and the shopping. His salary would hit their current account at the end of each month and Debbie would take care of the rest.

Much the same as now he reflected, except that now she begrudgingly allocated him what he needed to eek out some kind of existence.

It was this change in financial fortune that had made him come to discover how much toilet roll cost. He could recite the price of his shopping list by heart, except perhaps for the seasonal fluctuation in the price of bananas.

James passed the Scotsman's room again and heard a thick rattle of phlegm from behind the door. Quite revolting.
He entered his own room and quickly clicked the Yale lock shut. He detested that sickly cough.

The urgency of his actions had left him unbalanced and for a split second he'd forgotten where he was and now the lucidity had returned, he didn't want to turn around. He really didn't want to calculate the sum of his life by the inaccuracies of his surroundings and so fixed his gaze on the chips in the yellowing paintwork of the door and wondered who had put them there. But ah, now he was saved by some real distraction.

The title music for the Lake programme had begun and he needed to switch it over quickly and investigate the other channels. He turned and walked the narrow path to the wooden stand and picked up the mug of tea. Sitting himself at the edge of the bed he leant forward and pressed the stiff button of the programme changer with his thumb.

A repeat of *Seinfeld* that he'd watched the previous Friday, *Gourmet Cooking*, the fuzz of channel six, back to *Gourmet Cooking, Seinfeld, Ricki Lake* and another programme for pre-schools.

James turned off the television and sipped his tea. Perhaps he really would go down to *Parvs*. He could have a wander around the shops first and Monday was a market day so there was that to browse too.

He'd have a shower once he'd finished the tea.

Already the room was uncomfortably silent without the company of the television. James gulped at his drink to finish it and now all he needed to do was work out the viability of the trip before he set about getting ready.

He had fifty-two pounds left until pay-day which was eleven days away.

Bus fare to work and back: four pounds, leaving forty-eight. Launderette: two pounds thirty pence. Shopping, ten pounds, which would be especially tight this week as he would have to bear the brunt of a new can of deodorant and a fresh pack of razors. Canteen cost, one twenty-five times five... six-twenty-five, marvellous value really for a main meal. Cinema now: six pounds twenty pence. Sweets... say... two pounds. McDonalds, four pounds, although Adam sometimes went for a Fillet-o-fish and fries if he didn't want the toy in the Happy Meal, so say, five pounds to be safe. Pocket money two pounds, bus fare for them all, two pounds eighty. Phone calls over the ten days, although he'd be seeing them both for two out of the ten... so say, a pound. It didn't leave a lot.

James leaned back his head while he repeated the calculations grimacing at the inevitability of the sums remaining the same. He'd have ten pounds forty-five pence left once he'd made the deductions.

It wasn't enough to support the possibility of a few jars. He liked to have a little emergency money put by, at least ten pounds.

James laughed out loud at the next mental sum. Ten divided by ten equalling the enormous figure of one pound per day. It was going to have to be the sort of emergency you wouldn't dwell on once it had passed.

He swung himself back onto the bed and swore. What was he going to do with all of this day?

He toyed with the idea of turning the television back on. Alternatively, he considered buying himself a radio, just a smallish one that could pick up Radio Four. He doubted it would be very expensive, but then of course it would use all the cash he had.

But what about trying the library again? If he was lucky they might have got some new books in. It hadn't taken him long to exhaust the supply of anything vaguely readable, but it had been over three weeks since he'd last looked, so why not?

'Why not?' He asked his mirrored reflection.
James bounced up from the bed and set about gathering the clean underwear and wash-bag things from one of the wardrobes. He felt so much brighter now that he'd found a purpose to his day.

As he walked towards the shower room he even managed to reassert within himself a little confidence in getting that teaching position. Of course, he was getting on a bit, but they were crying out for teachers these days and what with all of his previous experience, however long ago it had been... besides, he knew he had to remain optimistic that life would get better.

He thought for a moment of the programme he'd seen recently on BBC2 regarding Philosophy and a particular bit concerning the butterfly effect. Apparently, all it might take was for a butterfly to flap its wings somewhere in the depths of the Amazon Rainforest and shortly after his bad luck would change.

Chapter 2 - Eve

It was Tuesday. They were all smiles when they huddled around her, Mr. Hepworth and his three young protégés'. No, students, that was the term he'd used and he'd introduced them so quickly Eve hadn't taken a single one of their names in, but she was sure it didn't matter.

'Good to see you again!' Mr. Hepworth said jovially holding out his hand.

Eve wasn't sure if she should have stood as she shook it, but there really wasn't the room so she stayed in the armchair feeling flush with indecision.

There was a bit of chit-chat about her settling in and a little joke about her escaping the bad weather but then the consultant's manner turned quite serious as he settled down to business.

For the sake of the young men Mr. Hepworth asked a series of rhetorical questions using the notes he'd taken during her appointment in his office.

'So, you underwent a lumpectomy just over seven years ago? Followed by a... six week course of radiotherapy? And since then you've been treated with Tamoxifen?'

He glanced briefly at the students and said 'ER positive' which Eve knew was right.

'You've been having regular mammograms since then, reduced to one a year for the last two years?'

He paused for a while, reading the notes to himself then he turned his head to face her and sighed before speaking a little softer than before.

'Unfortunately, the last mammogram and subsequent needle biopsy indicates the possibility of a new growth or re-growth and so we've taken the decision to have you in for both ultrasound and a CT scan and to perform a small procedure to remove a sample of your lymph glands for analysis, which I hope I explained well enough at our last meeting?'

Eve nodded compliantly to which the consultant responded with quite a broad smile.

'Thank heavens for that!' He quipped, 'I do feel I sometimes witter on endlessly without anyone having a clue at what I'm trying to say.'

The students laughed then, enjoying the joke, looking at one another with knowing eyes. Eve managed a faint smile but she was still anxiously waiting to ask her question.

'Okay then,' the consultant said eventually, as the laughter subsided, 'we shall see you again very soon with the test results.' He gave her one last smile and made to walk away.

Eve had meant to ask her question then but in her haste she merely blurted out a proclamation.

'I've got my son's wedding on Saturday.' She affirmed, feeling the redness back on her face.

Mr. Hepworth came to a halt, his face perplexed.
'We spoke about it at my appointment.' Eve continued.

The consultant still looked bemused, leaving Eve feeling quite stupid as the students followed her eyes.

Eventually she saw the flicker of recollection on his face.
'Ah yes!' he said grandly, 'of course!'

He quickly glanced back at his notes and sifted through the pages in search of the necessary information.
'You are booked in for theatre on Thursday morning, the CT scan should be done later this afternoon and the ultrasound will be done tomorrow morning... so yes, it shouldn't be a problem. Bearing in mind,' he added sternly 'you'll probably have to come straight back here in the evening.'

When they had gone Eve had got back into bed and began a crossword.
She felt so relieved that she'd had her hopes confirmed and now she wasn't afraid to think about the wedding. She pictured her dress and hat with pleasure and hoped the shoes she had bought wouldn't pinch her feet too much. She allowed her chin to slide into the palm of her hand which in turn was held rigid by an elbow fixed on the narrow table across her bed. Her mind was awash now of all manner of things that she'd managed to suppress until Mr. Hepworth had given her the okay.

She couldn't wait to see her boy in his tails and Rebecca, she just knew, was going to look spellbinding. Such a very pretty girl anyway, but in the dress she'd chosen, if it was anything like the way Rebecca had described it, it seemed there might be a few of them breathless in the congregation.

It was pointless carrying on with the crossword. Her mind was too absorbed with the wedding. Enjoy it she instructed herself. You can get excited now.

Of course, she didn't have much to do with the preparations. That was always the bride's mother's prerogative, though in all fairness she had been consulted about a lot of things, out of consideration more than anything else. Both Gill and Rebecca had been pretty thoughtful about that.

She put the crossword book back on the table and looked blankly around the ward.

It was far more pleasant than she'd hoped for. It was actually quite clean and no one looked particularly ill save perhaps the old lady in the next bed who seemed to have lay in exactly the same position since Eve had arrived. By the look on her face you could tell it wasn't a particularly comfortable position either. Most likely a stroke she thought.

The younger women over the way obviously knew each other quite well. Probably been in for a while she decided. They certainly didn't look ill. Two of them were always sauntering off to the main entrance in their garish nightclothes, smoking their cigarettes. Eve already knew she didn't like them. Especially the peroxide one whose name she'd overheard was Sam. Man's name, man's manners and god she was loud.

They were the only things Eve truly regretted about going NHS; the lack of privacy and having to put up with a bunch of fish wives.

The first time she'd gone private; own room with television, very good food, although, what with the operation she hadn't eaten much, but it was certainly an eye opener. Of course, that had all been paid for by the company's health insurance and now she was retired she found it too much of a waste to pay by her own means. Will had offered of course. Always ready with his cheque book, but she'd said to him she was sure the care would be just the same and at the end of the day she'd have the same consultant, private or NHS.

She suddenly felt a little wistful then, thinking about her youngest. She hoped Will could visit in the evening. It would be lovely to sit and talk about the wedding. Better still if he brought Rebecca along. They'd have a really good natter.

****

Friday at last but Eve felt awful, absolutely dreadful and that bloody old women had kept her awake for half the night as usual. Then the Sam woman had actually been a star. Sitting up, stroking the poor old girl while she sobbed, but of course as soon as she'd got back into bed she'd be howling again. God knows where the blooming nurses went.

She pondered Sam again. It just went to show how wrong you could be about people. She wouldn't want to be stuck in a conversation with her but she clearly had her heart in the right place.

Eve flinched as she adjusted her position in the bed. Her arm was really very sore and the pain killers were quite ineffective. She really did feel absolutely awful. She had been nauseas most of the night but had found it hard to sit herself up what with the dreadful soreness but by mid-morning she found herself dozing a little. It was quiet for once on the ward and the sun was pouring through the windows flashing sheets of light from the linoleum flooring that was quite sharp on the eyes so she kept them closed. Eventually she felt some level of comfort, though that could just have easily have been sheer exhaustion, either way she didn't even notice when she drifted into a deep nourishing sleep.

Suddenly it was Christmas and she was back in the old house. She could smell the pine needles as she entered the sitting room. It was barely daybreak and her new dressing gown reflected against the thick sheen of condensation that had always collected between the sash windows: A blur of emerald green.

Peter was there in his pyjamas crouched over the coffee table helping Matthew piece together the Meccano set they had bought him.

Billy sat cross-legged in the corner, all the booty from his pillow case spread neatly around him. He was wearing his new policeman's jacket and cap and chewing something chocolaty from his selection box.

'Oi young man!' she'd said jovially, 'you'd better not spoil your breakfast!'

Billy jumped up excitedly and began reeling off a list of everything he'd found. Too preoccupied to remember who had put them there. Brown saliva dribbled from the corners of his mouth.

'Tea darling?' she asked her husband.

'I'll do it!' Matthew exclaimed, rising from the floor.

'I'll help!' Billy had cried.

'You can't make tea Billy!' Matthew scolded.

'Yes I can!' Billy spat back, before a mad dash towards the door, each boy shoving past either side of her. They almost swept her off of her feet. She rolled her eyes up to the ceiling then down to Peter who was grinning between his stubble and showing all of his beautiful teeth.

****

Later, in the afternoon when she woke, she felt quite rejuvenated. The soreness was still there but it seemed much more bearable.

When she saw a nurse, she was going to ask if it was okay to drink some tea when the trolley came around. Her mouth felt completely parched.

She waited with eyes fixed on the doorway hoping to catch one of them as they busied by, then she heard footsteps, but instead of a nurse she was confronted by Mr. Hepworth and one of the young chaps who'd been in attendance previously.

Mr. Hepworth seemed quite solemn. He said hello of course, but then both he and his student pulled either curtain around the bed.

Eve made the gesture of pulling herself up from her prostrate position fully expecting the consultant to stop her in her tracks, raise the palm of his hand and tell her she was fine as she was, but he didn't. He let her struggle to a seated position leaving her sore and exhausted while he fiddled with a pen on the spring of his clipboard.

Mr. Hepworth sat down heavily in the armchair his mouth clamped shut. He took a deep draught of air through his nose. The notes before him made depressing reading, T4An3M1, which was just about as bad as they could be.

When she was quite upright, he looked up above his glasses and met her square in the eye.

'How are you?' He asked with a heavy sigh.
Eve assured him she was fine although still a little tender and still quite tired.
The consultant nodded sympathetically.

'We have your results,' he said, having taken a moment to choose his words. 'I'm afraid they're not at all good.'

Eve nodded discerningly. She'd been quite expecting it.
'Unfortunately, we can confirm a malignant growth on your breast which has metastasised or spread as it were, to other parts of your body. We've found it in both your lymph glands and your lung.'

There he paused for her to absorb the news.
'Is there any treatment?' She asked finally.
'Yes indeed.' He said gravely, 'However, due to the seriousness of your condition we will be unable to guarantee success.'

'And what sort of treatment is there?'
Mr. Hepworth explained the need to perform a mastectomy during which he'd remove the lymph glands then there would be a course of radiotherapy or chemotherapy on the lung depending on the size of the growth.

Eve had prepared herself for what she'd thought would be the worst, but the news of a secondary growth came as a real shock. She could feel the blood drain out of her but with determination she managed a dignified, if constricted, 'okay.'

'Now… with some further bad news regarding the operation,' the consultant continued reluctantly. 'It's extremely important that we tackle the problem as soon as possible and we have a slot for you, but unfortunately the slot is tomorrow morning.'

Eve's casing cracked. She could feel the tears roll down her cheeks.

'I'm terribly sorry.' The consultant said.

****

Sam thought Eve snooty, always had a bad smell under her nose. But watching her cry like that she couldn't help but pity her. She was obviously very proud, sitting there upright in her bed, staring into space, tears trickling down her face. Every now and then she'd dab them with a hankie. She could just as easily be peeling onions.

Sam left her to her tears for now. She knew from experience there wasn't anything you could do when people were like that even if you were close to them, let alone complete strangers.

Later in the evening the tears were gone. She looked sort of resigned now.

Sam had made up her mind to go and talk to her. Console her. She'd obviously had some bad news and from what Sam had seen she didn't have much family and definitely no husband. There was a sister she thought. Brought her in on her first day and visited a few times on her own. Then there was either a daughter or son and their other half. Probably he was the son 'cos he'd come without her tonight and had brought another bloke along. None of them ever stayed long.

Maybe she was just a cold bitch? Though on reflection that probably wasn't fair. Sam didn't know her. She might just be frightened; standoffish through fear. Either way Sam was determined to help her in some way if she could. Just a little chat maybe to let her know people were thinking of her.

All this sort of thing made Sam feel good. She'd found herself a bit in this rotten place, she was known for being good here; stroking

Olive to sleep in the middle of the night, sorting out some of the women's problems without being too full on.

Anyway, she took her chance coming back from a smoke. Eve was just sitting there staring into space. She smiled at her without any response but after she'd passed her she turned back like it was an afterthought.

'You alright now?' She asked softly.

Eve had tried to smile but then the tears had welled up in her eyes.

Sam grabbed her hand and gave it a squeeze.

'Come on darling,' she'd said, 'it probably ain't as bad as all that.'

Obviously, she didn't know at the time that it was as bad. Fucking bad it was. The poor cow was going to have her breast chopped off on the same day her only child was getting married.

He'd offered she'd said, her boy, offered to postpone the whole thing but she'd told him no; wouldn't want that she'd said. Breaks your heart Sam thought.

The woman who'd brought her, Penny was it? Was just her neighbour and no one was gonna be there when she had the op.

It does, she thought again; Breaks your heart.

****

It was Saturday and Eve lay in the dark. Eyes open looking up at the ceiling. Life's so strange she reflected. To think how down she'd been in the morning. It was bright first thing. Perfect wedding weather, but it hadn't lifted her spirits. Then of course Will had come early with Alan in tow, taking his best man duties very seriously.

Both she and Will were in floods of tears then, couldn't help it. Even Alan joined in. She could have quite easily lay down and died when they'd gone but then by some miracle everything changed.

A doctor she'd never seen before came along at midday and told her the news. The op had to be cancelled. He was so apologetic too.

'Honestly you couldn't have made me any happier.' She'd told him.

It was all a whirlwind after that. Sam dashed down to the main entrance where the telephones were and called Penny.

The nice young girl in the bed next to Sam did her hair for her and when Penny arrived they'd all helped her with her clothes and makeup and everyone was flattering about the outfit, genuinely too she thought.

Oh, and when it was time to go half the ward had got up to see her off; nurses too. It had made her feel so special.

Then of course there was the wedding. Oh god, the wedding. It was just so beautiful and then the speeches and the reception. Both boys did a lovely speech. More tears. Happy tears though.

Lots of people say that sort of thing about weddings she mused. 'Happiest day of your life.' but it really had been one of the happiest days of her life.

Penny was an absolute star staying off the wine all day so she could drive her back after racing to pick her up in the afternoon as well even though Alan had offered like the wonderful chap he was.

Only bit of sadness came when it was time to go. Will had broken down as he saw her off. Too much booze silly boy! He probably wouldn't remember half the evening. Rebecca was crying too but Eve told both of them to stop.

'No tears today.' She said. 'Today's a happy day.'

Chapter 3 – The Honeymooners

They had ordered a taxi from the wedding reception so no one would know where they were off to. No boisterous pranks would await them at the hotel. Will had even been careful enough to make the driver take them up to the gates of the lodge before instructing him where he was going.

Then on arrival at the Post house Will felt somehow deflated. Perhaps he would have wherever they had gone but the hotel exterior couldn't have looked more austere. He just hoped Becks wouldn't mind too much.

The reception area was surprisingly busy given the time of night and how it was the weekend. There were still quite a few guests sitting around the low tables drinking coffee from cheap crockery emblazed with the hotel's drab motif.

Will gazed at his bride who was shivering in her beautiful dress while he waited at the arrivals desk.

He wouldn't have been able to express how he felt just then, to see her leaning there with her slender arms wrapped around herself, but she was truly his now. How on earth had he managed that? He'd had his share of knocks in the past but look who he'd found to compensate.

A cheerless receptionist found their key and smiled dutifully through her tired make up as she handed it over.

They only had the one overnight bag as they were picking up the luggage from the apartment before they left for the airport. It was a good job Will thought as he squeezed the handle in frustration. No help had been offered.

It was completely his fault he rebuked himself as he collected his new wife and walked with her hand in hand back past the arrivals desk and towards the lifts. He should have made a concerted effort to find somewhere better. He was sure he could have done it if he'd really tried. The trouble was he'd been too laidback about the issue until it was too late. Neither he nor Becks had even guessed all the decent hotels would have been booked up so early. It still seemed ridiculously early when they'd began phoning around not to find somewhere good and for some stupid reason, he felt sure there would be a cancellation they could snap up... but there wasn't and now they were in this shitty salesman's rest that didn't even have a honeymoon suite. All the rooms were offered as standard.

They eventually found their room through the maze of corridors and fire doors and as first appearances went, they were both pleasantly surprised. It was bloody small but it seemed very well kept for what it was and the en-suite was actually quite plush.

'Oh, they've left us flowers.' Becky said brightly as she made her way towards the table.

Will had already observed the bottle of champagne in the ice bucket beside it and there was a small box of something else nice too.

'Oh look, a bottle of Champagne and chocolates.' Becky confirmed. 'With the compliments of Triton Group of Hotels.' She read excitedly from the card that she'd found perched against the basket holding the flowers.

'See it's really not so bad is it?' She enthused.
'There's some other stuff on the bed too!' Will pointed out eagerly.

They both made for the note at the top of the bedspread that lay on either side of two small boxes then glanced quickly at each other before spontaneously beginning a race to read it first, sniggering as they launched themselves across the bed, wrestling each other as they grabbed at it together.

Will used his superior strength to snatch it from her and turned to get away. Becky flung both arms around his neck in an attempt to pull him back and snorted loudly with her efforts but then came a small tearing sound.

'Oh no, my dress!' She cried letting go of him.
Will leapt up and scanned the delicate fabric while Becky clambered backwards feeling one of the boxes crush beneath her knee.

'Can you see anything?' She asked as she stood upright lifting her arms to examine the seams under her armpits.

Will moved round beside her for a closer inspection. They persevered for a couple of minutes but couldn't find any trace of a tear.

'I think it's alright.' He said finally.

'Mmm.' She agreed.

'You'd better take it off.' He suggested mischievously giving her one of his playful looks.

She smiled but changed the subject.

'What does the note say?' She asked.

Will had forgotten it was still there crumpled in his hand. He unfolded it.

'Oh fuck!' He cried as he recognised the handwriting.

'What!' Becky demanded in alarm.

'Alan.'

Will held up the message to show her.

At the top of the page Alan had written 'Don't panic!' Which he'd clumsily underlined.

The next line stated 'I haven't tucked you up I just wanted to prove once and for all that I'm cleverer than you.'

Further down the page on the right he'd written a note for Becky.

'Becky,' it said, 'flowers to keep when the real ones have died.' And under that a crude arrow pointing to the corner of the page. On the left he'd written a note for Will.

'Wills darling, you've got the ring so here's the sovereign to go with it (we'll make a real Essex boy of you one day). Anyway, I've seen your trading strategy and you can toss this now instead of having to beg for coppers.'

There was another arrow pointing to the opposite corner.

The newlyweds each reached over to the box where their arrow had once been pointing before their playful struggle.

Becky opened hers and found a gold brooch in the shape of a flower basket with semi- precious stones of different colours protruding from golden stems. Will tore open his box which was now crushed flat and sure enough there in a plastic sleeve was the sovereign glinting up at him.

'Silly git.' He said affectionately.

'Look, he must have spent a fortune.' Becky said passing the brooch over.

Will rolled it delicately between finger and thumb watching the bright colours flicker before him.

'You don't like this sort of thing do you?' He enquired.

'Oh I do! I love it!' She assured him.

'Good.' He sighed tossing the sovereign back onto the bed. 'I'd better do a full reccy now.'

Becky frowned.

'He said he hadn't done anything.'

'Him lie.'

Will pulled back the bedspread first then the blanket and sheets one at a time to find god knows what he wondered. He checked under the pillows and the pillowcases then under the bed. Becky made Will unzip her dress then picked up the overnight bag and headed for the bathroom.

'Be careful in there!' He called, 'cling film on the toilet... curry toothpaste...'

He waited silently for a while, half expecting to hear her shriek.

'I'm going to open the champagne.' He called without response. He drank a flute quickly then poured himself a second before flopping down onto the bed and slopping it over his suit.

'No decorum Billy Boy.' He mumbled to himself.

Once he'd finished the second glass, he stopped being concerned about Alan's schoolboy antics. They'd find them when they were caught up in them.

Even the sorrow for his mum that he'd been carrying at the back of his mind like a dead weight had dissipated and now he felt himself completely happy in the moment, there in that space and in their time. Nothing outside of it mattered. It was just him and Becks, his beautiful funny wife who made him ache with the love he felt for her. How could a loser like him be so lucky? He wondered in earnest, as he had so many times before.

When he'd got up to pour himself a third glass at the table the bathroom door opened. Becky appeared in the underwear she had selected for her wedding night. Her hair was wet and lank from the shower and the makeup had been wiped away.

Will found her more beautiful than ever.

'Wow.' He cooed.

She seemed awkward with her gesture but managed to smile her appreciation.

'No booby traps in there.' She said as she settled herself onto the bed.

'Trust me; Al's going to have the fire brigade or someone bang us up at three in the morning.'

'Well they'd better bang loud.' She said. 'I'm shattered.'

With her last comment Will thought it apt to take a shower himself but Becky stopped him.

'Let's finish the bottle,' she suggested, 'and will you pass over the chocolates please. I can let myself go now I'm married.'

They sat and shared the chocolates and smoked their cigarettes and talked about their day, what each one had missed and what they had shared together. They soaked in every little detail from one another's discourse feeling the warmth from the glow of what already felt like a fabled memory.

Both avoided speaking of his mother where possible. If she was mentioned they would flit to some other recollection as seamlessly as they could. Both felt each other's desire to dwell on that simple uncluttered joy for just a little bit longer.

Eventually, with the champagne drunk and the chocolate box empty Will rose to undress and have a shower.

Becky said his name solemnly and he turned towards her.

'Do you know,' she said softly, 'if Eve was my mum, I'd never forgive you if you made me go away on honeymoon.'

Will raised his hands as a question.

'We're staying.' She told him and she cradled him in her arms until his tears elapsed.

James had been fighting heroically against the urge to sob but finally he'd been beaten.

It was approaching six on a humid Friday evening and commuters with slick faces and crumpled clothes were swarming out of the train station and into bars or waiting their turn in the bus queues or the taxi rank.

James stood against the back of his bus shelter obscuring everyone's view of someone beautiful in the poster sized advert behind him. Each of the shelters that formed the town's main terminus were full with an array of hot and dishevelled travellers awaiting the chance to be crammed onto buses in the searing heat.

Bored car drivers sucked in the diesel and dust as they crawled past in the traffic absentmindedly scouring the queues for anyone or anything vaguely interesting to fill the wasted time.

If one were to choose a spot to have a breakdown in any sense of the word James was sure this would not have been it. So how mortified he now felt as the tears began to flow and the pathetic whimper he could no longer constrict rose from his throat like a sick dog's.

This was what his life had come to, the depths to which he'd plunged and now to compound his misery he was made to expose every frayed emotion to the introvert lines of fellow travellers who were no doubt primed toward any such distraction.

James closed his gritted eyes to the throng determined not to watch this new level of humiliation he had fallen down to being witnessed, but within moments of doing so there was the familiar vibrant groan of strained brakes and heavy metal as the next bus twisted around the tight corner.

There were a number of routes which started from his stop so he blinked his lids back open. Eighty-eight: two fat ladies in the mist. James wiped the moisture from his eyes to check again, the number had changed to eighty-six which wouldn't take him far enough in the right direction. He looked around at his audience and to his astonishment they were just as listless as before. The old woman to whom he'd earlier sacrificed his place on the bench was the only one who had returned a glance as she pulled her wheelie-bag onto the step of the eighty-six, the first of many to board.

Those that remained shuffled into the spaces vacated while James grimaced unsuccessfully in his attempt to stifle the next painful enunciation yet still no one seemed to pay him any mind.

James sought his reflection in the shop windows to ensure that he was really there. He found himself in an Estate Agent's display.

Now he understood.

It was an image of a man who had been quite tall but had learnt to stoop. Remnants of auburn hair remained but much had been diluted to varying shades of dirty orange that ebbed along the strands and ended in a dull grey. He wore his cheap rain jacket, more through fear of exposing his shirt than exposure to rain. James regarded its grubby canvas dolefully and even the reflection smelt of body odour.

Then there was the plastic bag. An even more fundamental expression of being poor he thought than wearing excessive cheap jewellery or expensive pumps.

The vision said it all: old, scruffy, ugly and boracic, beneath contempt.

James felt a fresh wave of self-pity storm out in disgust, leaving him choking back the tears again, yet why on earth should he care?

I'm an invisible man now, he conceded.

He looked down at the carrier bag he was holding which was struggling with its contents. He could probably drink one of the beers and no one would even raise an eyebrow. He knew the tins would soon become warm if they weren't drunk and he had nothing to chill them with again.

James placed the bag on the pavement then struggled to retrieve a tin from its snug neighbours.

The one-seven-four arrived and a decent proportion of the more affluent in the queue embarked then departed to the sound of a one can salute as James pulled the ring: tsk.

The lager was surprisingly cold and felt particularly gassy coming straight from the can. James had to stifle a belch. Having said that, did he really? he wondered. Would anyone hear it? Would anyone smell it?

He took another draught until there was nothing left to swallow and grimaced against the sharp pain at the back of his throat.

His reflection could have almost been smiling.
He carefully placed the empty can back in the bag and retrieved another.

Buses came and went as did the eighty-seven which was his ride home. He'd get the next one he decided and as he did so he gulped down the second can and bent down to retrieve the third.

The number of commuters in their suits had begun to diminish and the shelters emptied. James opened the fourth can theatrically.

A young woman came and sat at the bench beside him fussing shyly over her ugly baby in the buggy parked in front of her.

James watched her short denim skirt ride further up her thighs, legs to run away with he mused. He hoped she had somewhere good to go to and someone there waiting for her, but he sensed she didn't. Her face was so weathered and beaten which left him quite woeful.

The next can came and went in hopeless reflections.
Debbie in her own short skirts laughing discreetly at all of his jokes as he set the staff room ablaze with his own blend of cynical wit and pretentious eloquence.

She loved the way he spoke she said. It was one of the first things she'd told him. She was so young and vivacious then. So beautiful, then before he knew it, he was making love to the school secretary: All boobs and blond hair. He didn't even care who knew, was actually proud of it. He was almost daring someone to tell his first wife and save him the bother.

Now Debbie was three sizes larger and about as lovable as a pet tarantula and she'd even honed her evil powers to be capable of having him cry at bus stops.
'For heaven's sake change the subject' he muttered, it was no use getting depressed about it, although it wasn't easy not to.

He couldn't put to bed the wasted opportunity to start again. The firm's sudden relocation which he had actually managed to soak in and turn into something positive just for Deborah to put the dampeners on.

He'd done all the homework before he'd spoken to her knowing full well she'd be awkward, because she was always fucking awkward.

The firm were moving to Peterborough. He hadn't even been sure where it was to be honest, but he'd done his research. He'd spent three of the past four nights at the library on their computer finding everything out he needed to know about the town.

What had seemed daunting on Monday evening had become a gilt-edged opportunity by the Thursday and he actually thought, quite stupidly, he could bring her onto his side.

Was he ever going to learn?

Don't ever let it get you down he resolved trying to appear nonchalant for the benefit of the Estate Agent's window. Don't let her keep doing it to you. But he couldn't help it. Couldn't help playing that phone conversation over in his mind just one more time.

He'd begun so upbeat. Told her about the firm's plans, told her where Peterborough was and how far away it was from central London. Mentioned the relocation package he would get, hadn't even lied, although in all honesty it was hardly a large enough sum to merit any special caution away from her grasp.

'Where's all this leading to?' She'd interrupted with that bored distance she always had now whenever they spoke.

That was when James explained about the flats he'd read about. It was wonderful. One bedroomed flats were being advertised for rental for as little as two hundred and forty pounds per calendar month which was exactly the amount he was paying for the bloody awful bedsit he existed in now.

'It means the boys could stay.' He told her.

'What, the three of you in a poky one bed roomed flat?' Came the expected reply.

'Ah... I've thought about that,' he said cordially, hoping not to upset her by being a smart arse, 'I could get a sofa bed with the relocation money.'

43

There was a pause on the other end of the telephone while she no doubt contemplated her next derisive comment. James decided to get it over with quickly.

'There's only one important thing I need to clear up with you first,' he began sheepishly, 'I'm not going to be able to afford the train fares.'

He stopped purposely then knowing she'd rise to the bait. 'Don't think I'm going to pay!' She warned in her venomous tone.

'No, no,' he assured her calmly as his plan developed, 'I know you couldn't do that, of course not... all I was thinking was... perhaps I could travel down on the train on a Friday evening and borrow the car to take the boys to mine then back again?'

That was her cue to explain it would be too late in the evening on Friday to have them travel and then he would be seen to placate her by offering to travel down on a Saturday instead. The plan was going just as he'd hoped until that sudden moment when in a hare's breath it became derailed.

'No way!' She blurted. 'Sorry but you've got to be joking!' He had felt the aggression rise in his voice then which had totally blown any hope of negotiation out of the water.

'But I thought you only needed the car to ferry the boys around in?' He mocked.
'Well actually James, I need *my* car at the weekend!'
'*Our* car Deborah.' He reasoned, hating himself for using her full name which had always proved his anger.

'Erm, excuse me James, you seem to have lost your memory again? My car; end of story!'
There was a further pause then as he desperately tried to find something clever as a retort but she returned before it had formed.

'Right!' She stormed. 'Are we finished?'
'Fine!' He shouted spontaneously. 'I'll just have to see them once a month or whenever I can afford it!'

'Good idea.' She said dismissively. 'Goodbye James.'
He stood gasping for air in the phone box as the line went dead.

44

Doesn't matter, doesn't matter, doesn't matter he tried to assure himself now as he had tried to then, before opening the sixth and final can.

It was just a silly notion anyway. If she'd gone along with the car plan, he would still have struggled to afford the train fare for himself. Even if he had purchased the 'Super Advance Ticket' at only twenty-one pounds for a fifty-minute trip, as long as you booked it six years in advance! Then of course there was the petrol money and whatever premium, however tiny, would go onto Debbie's insurance which she was bound to make him pay. Bet your life she would. Just ten pounds extra per annum and she'd be standing there with her hand extended the very next time he went to pick up the boys.

She was like a vampire he surmised. Exactly that; like a vampire, bleeding him dry and literally sucking the life out of him. Taking his money, his children, his car, his home and now his little dream and she still had the cheek to use that attitude with him.

James sneered at the next oncoming bus. It wasn't his one but that didn't matter either way because he'd already decided. He desperately needed a leak and he desperately needed another drink and although he couldn't afford it, he was going on to the *Parvz* Bar.

Becky swept the tangled fringe from her brow and began walking again. She sensed it was useless to continue running. The station concourse was all but deserted except for a few in a similar predicament charging their way towards barriers that would only lead on to empty platforms.

She watched Will continue his run, turning his head at intervals to call after her, his words rebounding inaudibly against the locked shutters of the fast food outlets.

A digital clock high above her flicked its last digit from a seven to an eight which confirmed the race was truly over as the final train was scheduled to depart at twelve forty-seven.

She looked down from the clock and found Will further in the distance. Stationary now but arms flailing like a lunatic directing an anguished cry of disgust toward the train as it slipped out of the station.

Now she had to watch with some trepidation as Will's attention switched to the ticket man behind the barrier; Just a little Asian guy with a big bushy beard and an oversized cap. God only knew what crap Will was spouting at him.

Whatever it was, the poor man had obviously heard it countless times before because if body language was anything to go by, he didn't seem the least bit phased.

A few months previous she might have found the scene comical in a way, she'd had enough to drink herself and watching Will standing there like an idiot, all red-faced slurring gibberish as the man starred back with a blank expression from somewhere behind his beard would have probably been hilarious. She could have given him a real slating in the morning and he would have been sheepish and embarrassed and then they'd just have a laugh about it.

That wouldn't happen now though. Not since his mum had died. He seemed to have had a sense of humour failure since then. She was sure she would feel different about the world if and when it happened to her and she'd be more than a little bit freaked out as well but to be honest Will was seriously beginning to go off the rails. His drinking was worse than it had ever been. He was getting into all sorts of scraps. His work was suffering as well according to Alan, or at least according to what Alan had told his other half.

It was still impossible to fathom how badly he'd taken it about his Mum. She couldn't get him to talk about it. Obviously, it was awful the way she went, ebbing away in her bed in all that pain so she knew it must have crushed him? Mustn't it?

Becky didn't even want to ever properly think about what it would be like when either of her parents went; she couldn't even begin to imagine it. Her mum was her best friend in the world other than Will.

Eve and Will were different though, like a proper old-fashioned mother and son relationship. They didn't even seem that close to be honest. He never visited her that often and he might only phone her once a week and that would be over almost as quickly as it had begun; Becky wondered if he regretted not showing her how much he loved her and perhaps that was why? Perhaps he felt he couldn't get all emotional over her death when he didn't really show what you might have expected him to when she was alive? She didn't know, really, she didn't; although in his defence he was with her every chance possible when she was dying and besides, Becky thought, wasn't a relationship meant to be a two way street?

Didn't matter now though did it? The important thing now was whatever was going on in Wills mind she'd have to live with, with him, ride it out and hope he didn't do anything too stupid in the meantime.

At the end of the day, however long he was going to fight it for, he needed to grieve.

So, he'd shed a few tears the afternoon she died and he'd wiped a few more on his sleeve at the funeral. But other than that, he seemed to be blanking everything out.

Becky totally expected him to get emotional on the day they'd cleared out Eve's little house, his own house for so many years, but they were in and out in a couple of short hours. He stayed focused and business like the whole time.

He only let her go with him because Penny, the neighbour, had volunteered herself to help and he didn't want to be stuck on his own with her.

Becky couldn't help think it would have been useful if he'd slowed down and soaked in a few memories but he was straight into Eve's bedroom and emptying out the mounds of paperwork he knew she had tidied away at the bottom of her bedroom wardrobes. He wanted to find the bills and contacts to have her utilities turned off and any subscriptions stopped. All of the essential stuff that needed doing.

Penny and Becky had been left to pack up his mum's clothes and personal effects into the plastic bags Becky had brought with her ready for the charity shops.

Will didn't want to keep any of the fine china and crystal Eve had on display in the glass cabinets in her living room. He wanted Penny to take the lot and when she tried to insist on him having them, he threatened to give it all to charity. A bit too aggressively for Becky's liking but Penny was as good as gold and told her in private that she'd store it all away for them until Will had time to think about it some more.

Will said he'd found quite a few personal bits among the mounds of paperwork as he sifted through. Old Christmas cards and one or two letters from old friends. Some with return addresses and he'd mentioned that he wished he'd done the clear out earlier so he could have let those people know about the funeral. There hadn't been many there. No relatives at all, which wasn't a big surprise given how Eve had cut herself off from them all after her husband had gone awol.

So, it just left Penny and her other half and one or two other elderly ladies that Becky had never met before to witness the proceedings. Needless to say, the wake was a truly sombre occasion which reflected, if she was being honest, a fairly sombre life.

None of the ladies drank even a drop of alcohol. It was orange juice and lemonade they used to wash down the few nibbles of sandwiches they'd eaten. One old dear just stuck to a glass of water which was only to sink an extraordinary amount of pills at an exact time in the afternoon.

Fortunately, Alan was there god bless him. Best man and best mate in every way. He obliged in keeping Will company while they both sunk a gallon or so of Guinness.

Only Penny's other half could be cajoled into drinking anything strong and that, Becky thought, was no more than a pint of some ale concoction. Sipped it he did until Penny and the other ladies let a respectable amount of time pass before they made their leave and left just Will and Al propping up the bar while Becky waited patiently for them and watched the landlady clear away so much untouched food.

'I had to give them a decent spread.' Will had said in his defence. Becky supposed that he had wanted to show that Eve had left a legacy: The successful son with the nice car and a tailored suit giving them all a decent spread.

That was that it would seem as far as Will was concerned, that whole chapter of his life now over.

Still at least he'd brought home quite a lot of stuff from Eve's wardrobe, random family stuff.

Becky thought it was really sad to see how surprised Will had been that she'd kept those things that you'd take for granted a mother would keep.

There was him and his brother's old school books and reports and various cards both her children had made for her, quite a few old Polaroid's too that Will had no memory of. There was a lovely black and white one of the two boys when they were really young sitting next to each other, all smartly dressed with little shirts and ties, very sweet... course Will was too young to remember what for.

He even brought back a great heavy box thing covered in red leather. He said there'd been an old gramophone player inside when he was a child but now it was full of birth certificates and various other registration forms, nothing worth looking at he had said even if he was careful about re-locking it.

Hopefully in all that lot, there would be something that may spark him into mourning.

Heaven knew she couldn't put up with this sort of nonsense forever.

Will turned to her as she approached. He had got himself so worked up he actually had tears in his eyes.

'Will, can you stop it!' She snapped.

'What?'

'Can you please stop shouting at that poor man?'

'Listen,' he slurred while trying to focus on her face, 'I was just asking why they always let the last train go bang on time when they know there's people running to catch the fucking thing.'

His anger began to recede when he'd finally managed to see the full extent of Becky's disapproval. His own expression quickly changed to bewilderment as he realised she wasn't at all supportive of his argument.

'But how often are they delayed?' He whined. Becky shrugged wearily.

'How often are these fucking trains late!' He roared, turning his attention once again to the platform attendant.

'Please Will!' Becky pleaded.

'Always fucking late.' He continued, a good deal subdued, yet still jabbing his index finger in the direction of the small gap between the man's cap and beard.

Becky tugged at the untidy swathe of hair that had fallen back over her eyes then began to knead it gently into her forehead with the palm of her hand.

'Please,' she uttered feebly, 'please can we just go home?'

Will was just about to part his lips in preparation of his next outburst but thought better of it. He stood instead in sullen silence as his mind switched to more practical thoughts; A place to get a cab. Would the rank still be open he wondered? But of course not, the rank closed down in line with the station. Then he remembered the taxis that always lined up out on Bishopsgate until really late. He turned to his wife to tell her and noticed how drained she looked and suddenly felt pangs of guilt for keeping her out for so long.

He slowly moved toward her and gently lifted her chin with a forefinger. She looked dolefully up at him.

'What Will?' she asked dismally.

He wrapped his arms around her slender shoulders and pulled her gently toward him.

'Let's just go home.' She mumbled, letting her head rest against his chest for a moment; then she was pushing him away feebly with her hand, eager to begin the journey home.

'I'll go and get a cab.' He said soothingly, releasing her and within a moment he was bounding up the short flight of escalators toward street level.

Becky turned with a faint smile for the poor platform attendant hoping it might make some amends for her husband's behaviour before following him wearily into the night.

Outside the street was stark. The hordes of thousands that had packed the pubs and bars around the station had finished their drinks on mass and taken their fast food and high spirits home with them. Wrappers and crushed cartons lay on the quiet pavement to mark their passing.

The lights were out in the fried chicken restaurant opposite and a solitary waiter stood guard in his bow tie and grubby waistcoat behind the hatch of the all-night café a few doors down. The feeling of solitude leapt from the abandoned office space surrounding her. She shivered in the still night air.

To Becky's relief she finally spotted Will further along the street before a whole row of taxis. He was talking to a group of men huddled together around the first vehicle. Fortunately, they all looked like cabbies, drinking coffee out of polystyrene cups.

They seemed to be enjoying a quiet joke with Will and now they were all watching her approach.

However sloshed she was, she still couldn't help feel terribly self-conscious of all the eyes that greeted her as she joined them. She wrapped her suit jacket tightly around her.

The gentle laughter had almost dried up now and only Will was left doing the talking.

Becky had assumed he was trying to haggle them down. The sort of thing he could brag about at work to Alan and the other traders, making the cabbies squabble over what looked like the last fare of the night; but once in earshot she realised she was completely mistaken. Will was actually moaning at them all. Mumbling really, but moaning just the same.

'You guys are unbelievable' he said, shaking his head with dismay.

The cabbies with some subtlety had managed to turn slightly away from him before he had even finished and within an instant were making small talk among themselves.

'What's the matter? Are you guys afraid of earning money?' He complained, a good deal louder now.

Becky tactfully slipped her arm through his knowing what his temper had been like of late.

Will turned to her exasperated. 'Can you believe they want a ton to take us home!' He ranted.

'How much is a ton?' She asked blinking wildly to shield herself from his next outburst.

'A hundred quid!'

'No!' She gasped incredulously.

'Yeah!' He assured her, throwing his voice for the benefit of the group who had by now formed a circle with their backs turned.

'A hundred fucking quid for an hour's work!' He cried.

'I don't even earn that sort of money!' He spat which Becky found both unnecessary and unhelpful.

The couple stood rooted for a short while somehow expecting a response then Becky felt Will stagger backwards a little and had to steady him with all of her remaining strength.

She suddenly felt quite nauseous with fatigue and perhaps all the wine she'd drunk, it was enough to conclude that she needed the comfort of her bed as quickly as possible and at whatever the cost.

'Let's just get in one.' She suggested meekly.

Will glared at her furiously.

'No fucking hope' he said and shook her arm away from his.

'Well I'm not getting a bloody night bus!' She shouted.

'Fine!' He retorted, backing further away from her.

'Get a cab... I'll see you at home. Go on fuck off!'

Becky watched him turn and walk heedlessly away from her, stumbling over a bag of rubbish in his eagerness to escape. She was grabbing at her hair again and pummelling her aching temples.

'Will!' She called finally as his figure began to dissolve into the blue haze of the distance. She watched him all the way down to the corner that would take him around to Houndsditch, waiting fretfully for him to disappear altogether but then suddenly he paused.

Becky shook her head in disbelief.

Doesn't have a clue where he's going, she thought. He seemed to be searching in his pockets now. Found whatever it was and was leaning forward.

The bastard had only stopped to light a cigarette she realised with disgust as she saw the flame flicker.

Thought he'd be gone now but he wasn't. He'd turned again and was walking back toward her and with some purpose too.

What a sodding waste of time that had been she thought. She was beginning to seethe a bit to be honest, but she'd let it go for tonight. She wasn't going to scare him off again now; but tomorrow, she was definitely going to have words.

He was still grim faced as he approached her, then he was pulling her gently by the arm.

'Come on,' he said assertively, I've thought of something.'

'Where are you taking me?' She groaned after Will had marched her for fifty yards.

He nodded up towards the building beside them. Becky snatched her arm back from his clutches.

'Stop mucking me around!' She snapped, bringing herself to an abrupt halt.

'I'm not.' He tried to assure her.

'Then where are we really going?'

'There... *really.*' He said with another nod upwards. 'The Great Eastern.'

Becky regarded the building with some disdain. She looked through the darkened windows at the silhouettes of tables and chairs and perhaps the brass frame of a bar.

'You want us to stay here?' She asked in bewilderment.

'Why not?'

Becky knew the Great Eastern Hotel by reputation. She'd never stayed there herself but she'd heard her share of illicit tales about the place. It was even said you could rent the rooms by the hour.

'I'm sorry,' she said sternly, 'I'd sooner walk home then stay in a rundown knocking shop.'

'No, no, no,' Will corrected her then grinned, 'it's all changed. It's been totally renovated now. It was taken over by Conran and some big American chain. They've spent millions doing it up.'

Becky considered this new information sceptically. It certainly didn't look any different from the outside. The Victorian façade remained, sending great elevations of ugly red brick hurtling towards the skyline and the lanceted windows still reminded her of a Dickensian workhouse.

'It'll cost a lot more than a cab fare.' She convened.

'I don't care.' He said petulantly with the taxi drivers fixed in his thoughts.

'And we haven't got any clothes for the morning, any deodorant, toothbrushes... anything.'

'Oh, come on!' Will moaned impatiently. 'They'll have all that sort of stuff in there. Or at least shower gel and toothpaste and what have you. They're bound to have those little complimentary tooth brushes, even that Triton place did... So, we won't have clean underwear, so what? All we'll be doing in the morning is getting on an empty train and going home.

Becky pondered the idea a little while longer, searching her head for further obstacles to the plan although she couldn't quite rationalise the reason why. After all, she was exhausted and far too fuddled to care about the morning or fresh knickers or anything else for that matter. Perhaps it was just the drink making her feel obstinate she decided. However, she couldn't resist one final hindrance.

'What about deodorant then?'
Will squinted in contemplation for the answer.

'Don't you carry some in your handbag?' He asked.
'But that's only a roll-on.'

'Oh, for fuck sake Becks!' He groaned and as he did so she couldn't stop her dry lips parting defiantly into a glimmer of a smile.

'Well you can't use it.' She said. 'I'm not having all of your armpit hair stuck to it.'
'Fine, I'll go without... so does that mean?'

'Alright then!' She conceded. 'But don't start swearing at anyone and playing up in there!'

Will stretched out his hand, which she took with feigned indifference.
They began walking again, turning slowly into Liverpool Street itself.

Shortly after they passed a large black door with an elegant framed restaurant tariff at its entrance. Becky could just make out the two largest words at the top of the page which she unwittingly read aloud.

'The George.' She announced.
'I've eaten there.' Will remarked as they continued on their way. 'We took some Koreans there.' He recalled. 'Me and Ken; they wanted to try English but afterwards we took them to the Chinese Karaoke.' He reflected fondly.

Will and Becky passed a second stylish restaurant in the same building, this time Japanese.

'See I told you they'd done it up.' Will reaffirmed.
Becky didn't feel inclined to reply.

They reached the revolving doors that lead into the hotel foyer. Will slipped through first, sensing Becky's reluctance to lead.

The marbled foyer seemed quite stark but for the two small exotic trees set in tubs on either side of the doorway and the short reception desk, the function of which was announced with a garish neon sign above it.

Becky hung back as Will spoke quietly to the two receptionists. There was a brief period of inaudible banter where he made both girls giggle and then his credit card appeared and finally one of the girls produced a key fob.

Will beckoned his wife over, waving the fob happily and within a moment they were across the lobby and into the deep silent lift that raced them towards their room.

As soon as they were inside Becky swept backwards onto the bed with a contented groan. She kicked her shoes onto the floor. 'Bliss.' She sighed.

Will removed his jacket and hung it carefully on the back of a desk chair. He surveyed the room with satisfaction then let himself fall gently onto the bed and by her side.

They lay there breathing heavily and unable to stir. Will glanced sideways at his wife whose eyes had closed. If he had thought of turning off the light before he lay down, he was sure they could both have happily fallen asleep as they were. It was a supreme effort on his part to raise himself again and begin to discard his shoes and crumpled clothing across the floor.

'Becks,' he said wearily, 'get undressed darling.'
Becky had no desire to move at all and would have stayed prostrate where she lay if Will hadn't have pulled her up by an arm. He helped her remove her jacket and then the trousers before hanging them both neatly in a wardrobe. Becky managed the rest herself while Will trudged arduously toward the bathroom to use the toilet

and clean his teeth with his index finger and the tiny tube of complimentary toothpaste provided.

By the time he'd returned Becky had found her way under the covers and had curled herself into a foetal position. He turned off the light and slipped between the cool linen sheets. He could feel the soft cold soles of her little feet caress his calves and thighs before quickly moving off; then she breathed goodnight and within a moment she was asleep.

With one last effort Will dragged himself onto his back and stared contentedly into the darkness, enjoying the firmness of the bed.

He hoped the day's disasters at work wouldn't wake him before morning which had often been the case lately. But his time to ponder was brief; within a minute his wife's steady breathing had coaxed him to join her in slumber.

It was almost two hours later when Becky climbed from the bed and made her way as quickly and quietly as possible to the bathroom with the notion of being sick.

She had almost been rugby tackled to the floor by Will's carelessly discarded trousers which had completely exasperated her considering the effort he'd made to keep his jacket smart: but she'd managed to keep her expletives to a whisper for fear of waking him.

She crouched for some time over the porcelain bowl but the vomit wouldn't rise although she could feel it whirling inside her. Fatigue overcame her and she found herself on her knees with her arms stretched across the rim of the seat. Her head propped between them and toward the abyss.

It was the chill that woke her again. The muzziness had gone but now she was shivering with cold and her dry teeth chattered. She tried to pull herself up only to find that both legs had gone quite dead under her body. There was nothing else to do but wait for the circulation to return.

Some lucidity returned during the vigil and she silently cursed all the ingredients that had helped shape her present situation. Binge drinking, skipped meal, drunkard of a husband, greedy cab drivers. Most of all she berated herself. This sort of behaviour should be in the past. She was a married woman now and she should be discouraging Will from this kind of performance rather than giving it credence.

When the tingling had subsided and enough feeling had returned to her legs she crept unsteadily into the bedroom, avoiding all the obstacles now that her eyes were accustomed to the dark.

A fresh wave of nausea, though thankfully much milder, echoed inside her as she slipped back into bed. She cussed her feeble inability to stick her fingers down her throat as she lay flat in the hope of sleep's return or a fresh upsurge that would bring her suffering to an odious yet longed for conclusion.

She was still shivering under the blankets and her head had begun to throb. All she wanted was just a little more rest.

At that moment Will shot up beside her.
What now? She thought.

Will groaned a deep woeful groan and began clawing at the bedclothes.
'For Christs sake stop being so bloody selfish!' She snapped as she raised herself to scorn him further, but his ashen face suddenly frightened her.

'Will!' She shrieked in alarm and he turned to her with eyes bulging.
Becky watched the man she knew so intimately draw in the air with what seemed like terror then let out a high-pitched wail. In that moment it was as if she were looking at a stranger.

'Will!' She shrieked again. 'Will... you're frightening me!'
She grabbed quickly for his hands and made them stop; but now his eyes began to reel and he shuddered.

Becky could only watch horrified, yet within a moment Will's eyes were still again and she could see his pupils adjust to the darkness. He was swallowing hard and she could tell he was trying to talk but his speech was constricted by his attempt at haste.

'Slow down.' She said soothingly, releasing a hand and stroking her palm gently against his forehead.

Eventually his perseverance won through and he was able to be heard.

'Jesus, I had a horrible dream!' He exclaimed.

'Oh my god! You scared the shit out of me!' Becky snapped with relief.
She glided her hand back down across his arm still stroking him tenderly as she shifted herself recumbent again.

'Jesus that was horrible.' Will reiterated rubbing his own hand over his furrowed brow and through his spiky hair, feeling a flood of perspiration as he did so.
'What a shitty dream.' He continued.

As his eyes adjusted further to the blue darkness of the room, he thought he could see a mischievous twinkle in Becky's eye and with a slight pang of irritation he could see that she was smiling.

'Oh, don't take the piss.' He whined, the effect of which only made her slide into a fit of giggles.

'Nasty piece of work.' He uttered jovially, realising how ridiculous he must have sounded before.

Becky made an effort to constrain herself.
'It was only a nightmare.' She teased.

Will grabbed her by the wrists and lifted her before pushing her back onto the pillows.

'Just a nightmare eh!' He growled. 'Well you wait till I tell you all about it... you should've seen this old man...'

'Please... not now.' She begged. 'I'm having a bit of a nightmare myself. I've been trying to throw up for ages and I desperately need more sleep.'

She leant across and kissed him gently on the cheek. 'Please let's sleep.' She whispered.

It was probably no longer than fifteen minutes before the acid in Becky's stomach had settled and she was able to drift glassy eyed into an uneasy state of repose. Will lay with his head against the soft linen of his pillowcase and watched her; glad to see her resting.

He thought about the nightmare for a while then dismissed it as nothing more than the consequence of sleeping in a strange bed in a strange room.

It probably hadn't helped that the exterior of the building reminded him of some sort of Dracula's castle.

He couldn't imagine he was going to get any more sleep himself so he'd content himself by lying there peacefully with his eyes closed, then at eight in the morning he found himself being shrugged awake.

Fear me not!

I be above you once again but only by illusion and cannot harm you though I am a true man of flesh!

Pray then forgive my coarse appearance for I have been bled head and neck to free my body of ill humours.

Though I be sure my visit doth clearly vex you sir by the way your face doth contort I am truly sorry to make such an unwanted intrusion yet you will find by my discourse presently how urgent my need be to find accomplices in a task of such magnitude it may yet mean the saving of mankind should we succeed.

Forgive also then my weeping for I am so deeply gladdened to come upon you for a second time which may yet finally lead to my burden being shared.

I must begin then at haste before your conscious self does awake and cast me out once more.

Just brief descriptions that describe myself and so to assure you of my good character contrary to how I now appear before you.

I am a gentleman of the best quality and intellect sir despite appearance that present circumstances have bestowed upon me and have been a merchant of the finest wines from both France and Spain and hath served the Court and all of London for many a year before this sorry incarceration.

Yes, I am imprisoned sir! Not such a place where rogues must serve a punishment but a place where those judged not fit of mind must be locked away lest the truth be conveyed to all and a solution be gathered from a common effort.

Indeed, I have the worst tidings for I have witnessed such dreadful conflagrations upon London. Two dreadful episodes of devastation I have seen but yet a third I fear hath left the city razed.

I speak to you from the year 1663 sir, it may be more than your wit may allow you to believe yet I must coax you my way with the proof of these dreadful discoveries.

There will be a great fire soon sir just as Mother Shipton did prophesise and I know not even of my own fate or that of my family only sure I have seen the flames sweep from building to building from there by London Bridge and down to the Three Cranes thus destroying the Vintrie Wharf and with it all of my warehouses and goods. No one more to help than nightsoilmen and fishmongers and that after they did move their own stalls and belongings.

It will be proof to you sir! A calamity of such magnitude that it will surely be recorded by the aldermen and those of the church that will mourn the final passing of Saint Paul's which roof I did see sink upon itself.

With what length of time I cannot calculate but I did see the city rebuilt from the ashes to a size and of a beauty I could not have foreseen. Buildings tall and all of brick and stone, the streets widened in all places for carriages to pass on both sides there together.

Then what if I tell you of those carriages sir? Horseless all! Ponder then, could I have imagined such science without being witness to it?

But then I did see a greater marvel most unnatural to me that did fill me with both terror and awe. The sky adorned with winged carriages that man hath made to mimic the flight of birds. Few at first and passing high but then they came in flocks arriving by moonlight to swoop down upon the town to drop their bombs as if they were but laying eggs.

Devastation sir!
Each blast did light the night sky and scare fires were cast all around. Whole structures crumbled in their wake and streets collapsed as one so that I could scarce believe a single building or soul would remain. Night after night they came, the cannon below useless to deflect them.

Dark days indeed which I have no doubt you would have been schooled the details of, yet all this I did see and then with such relief the mirth of the crowds when the attacks did cease.

Am I then a madman or can you now be ready to learn from further disclosure of London's fate?

I beseech you to heed my warning and to act upon it with your best endeavour.

Alan always looked so bloody dapper. Crisp shirt, pressed suit, polished shoes: didn't matter what hedge he'd been pulled through or what bar he'd been thrown out of he was always at his desk early, looking smart and able.

The only tell-tale signs that he may have been burning the candle at both ends would be a slight redness in those dark eyes that every woman seemed to go weak for.

Will didn't mind most of the time. He was his best friend after all; he'd even been his best man for Christ's sake and he'd *really* been the best man when his mum was dying and everything he'd done for him afterwards. Will would never forget that.

That was why he couldn't help berate himself for even that slight twinge of resentment. He knew Al didn't deserve it.

It was only that he'd seen himself in the lift mirror on the way up and he looked like shit and felt even worse but Alan was at his desk like always, bright as a button, smoothing back his curly black hair and grinning from ear to ear.

The banter had already started. No doubt he'd be all set to have a friendly dig about Friday's cock-up.

'Shag!' Alan greeted him loudly from across the rows of desks. Will hung his crumpled raincoat on his designated hanger and made his way uneasily to his work station.

'Oh dear.' Alan grimaced as he folded the tabloid he'd been reading. 'Another one of those weekends was it?'

Will rolled his blood shot eyes in silent assent then slumped into his chair and stared forward in solemn contemplation.

The Reuters and Bloomberg screens blinked intermittently before him.

Will knew he could lift this feeling of dread he had again if he could just focus on the job and relax. Focus... and... relax he told himself. All he needed to do was find a steady breathing pattern.

Alan left him to it. Unfolded the paper again and went back to reading a disturbing article about the latest Taiwanese bid for independence.

Eventually Will managed to get his breathing under control again, perhaps the distraction of the Reuters had helped, but whatever the reason, he wished he'd managed it as easily on the train journey in.

Still wasn't sure how he'd saved himself from a heart attack when the train had ground to a halt for the best part of ten minutes as it approached Limehouse.

Couldn't catch his breath he was so wound up and god only knew what the woman next to him had thought, he was fidgeting so much as he contorted himself to gasp the air. Next he was trembling and then the palpitations had started. Worse was when the real pains began shooting through his chest and he started sweating, really, really sweating. Sweating and trembling and still he couldn't breathe.

Then thankfully the fucking train had finally started moving again and he had somehow recovered but for the numbness and tingling in his fingers.

'So how was your weekend?' He managed to muster with some considerable effort for his friend.

'Oh, we're talking now are we?' Alan quipped.

'Please mate,' Will pleaded, 'don't pick on me today: I'm dying.'

'Oh, Will's baby, when do I ever pick on you?' Alan cooed affectionately.

'Just do me a favour then mate will ya? Come for a drink at lunchtime.'

'It's not even nine o'clock on a Monday morning!' Alan said aghast.

'I never said right now, did I? ...I said lunchtime.'

Alan frowned his reluctance.

'I hate drinking this early in the week.'

'I really need a hair of the dog Al.' Will pleaded.

'Why don'tcha just take some of the totty from accounts?'

'Because Derek gives me a hard enough time when I bring them back pissed on a Friday.' Will responded plainly. 'God knows what he'd say to me today.'

Both men scrutinized one another for a time in wilful silence.

'I'll tell you what Will,' Alan proposed at last, 'you sort out this Delta thing from Friday and I'll go for a drink with you.'

'Nothing to sort.' Will answered bluntly.

Alan raised a doubtful eyebrow in his direction.

'I've already had it out with Clive.' Will said defiantly.

'Fine, but you haven't filled the hole yet have you?' Alan pointed out abruptly.

'Soon as the market opens.' Will tried to assure him.

Alan shrugged his opinion at this last announcement and turned his attention back to the paper.

'Listen, Clive's happy to fill it at market!' Will said with growing irritation.

'Course he is,' Alan chuckled, 'but the market's on the up son. You'll never get the offers before lunchtime... in fact you'll be lucky to have 'em by Friday lunchtime.'

'We'll just have to see wont we!' Will retorted with what he hoped appeared an air of smugness if only to disguise his true thoughts on the subject. He could barely summon any optimism if truth be told.

Alan sat quietly amused and began to peel the first of a variety of snacks he had made a habit of consuming throughout the course of his working day.

Will waited impatiently for the hands of his watch to creep towards the hour and just before the market opened he wasted no time in calling the first broker.

'I'll take all front month offers at market.' He mumbled into the receiver then immediately ringing off to call a second broker.

Alan was watching the opening bids on the screens before him. He grimaced sympathetically as he caught Will's eye.

'On the bright side,' he spluttered, swallowing the last mouthful of a banana, 'you were right all along son: we got a Contango market!'

Will knew very well that he'd been right. His first really successful hunch that whole fucking year and the first time in too long that the demand for sugar had significantly exceeded supply. He had had the foresight to build a large position on the futures market to sell when the price reached its peak and of course he'd taken the whole position in his own speculative book which meant the profit it realised would have helped improve the size of his bonus enormously.

He should have known nothing that straightforward was ever going to be straightforward. It was just this sort or market that was going to test the systems and procedures and sure enough it came to light that the option deltas hadn't been calculated properly.

Now the firm found itself exposed. Could be offset of course against all he'd built.

All weekend he'd prayed he could fill enough of the position before the price really leapt rather than use everything he had to rectify the obligations the company had with its third parties. Though just a glance at the screens at this early stage was enough to suggest it was going to be impossible.

As he watched the price steadily climb Will once again seethed at Clive's unfairness in forcing him to handle all of the hedging for the physical traders and keep up a good spec account *and* police the guys in the back office.

Of course, in Friday's spirited meeting Clive had been quick to point out that as far as he understood, half the reason Will had been promoted from back office to futures trader was to use his experience to keep a careful check on every function which included the p&l reporting.

Will had countered, with a barely veiled rage, that it was ridiculous to be expected to check something as fundamental as the deltas hitting the position. He'd actually sworn in his frustration, took everyone aback, himself included, which was probably why Clive had made the concession of letting him fill at market if he could; although in all honesty they both knew how empty the gesture had been: yet, until this morning Will had at least hoped he could claw something back.

But looking at the screens again it was already clear he was going to be left with nothing and that was if he was lucky. It had to move for him soon or else he could see the book going into the red as the price reached an early high, dipped then rose again.

At just past eleven Alan looked up at Will from the waste paper basket he'd hunched himself over to unfoil the Kit Kat he was about to make disappear. He didn't want to say anything now. The market had just gone up and up, exceeding any sort of expectation he'd had. It finally dawned that Will was going to miss out on an awful lot of money.

Will looked back at Alan with a resigned expression and slowly began to speak.

'So, if I transfer the position over, are you still going to buy me a drink?'

Of course he would, thought Will. He didn't really need to ask and the good thing was that Alan wouldn't dare tease about anything work related now so Will would be free to talk about the nightmares that were beginning to freak him out. Alan would make sense of them or at least put them into some sort of perspective. Will certainly knew he needed help with perspective: he'd just missed out on the best part of ninety grand and the only real concern he had... and he had to stop and wonder at himself... was that he'd be able to talk about and hopefully, please god, get rid of those stupid bloody nightmares!

'Better?' Alan asked as Will placed the empty whisky glass down onto the bar.

'No.' Will replied glumly.

It was going to take a hell of a lot more than a large whisky to get away from death's door.

Alan sipped at his pint as he pondered a way of encroaching on the subject. It wasn't going to be simple. This was easily the biggest personal loss he'd heard of since the personal performance scheme had been implemented.

Well that's true, it suddenly occurred to him. At least he'll have the sympathy of the desk. If we were still on the share scheme they would have hung him up by his balls and I'd probably have helped them.

Oh, another thing: if it didn't affect his PPS would Clive have stood such a big loss?

It wasn't as though Will had been doing it this year.

Okay, fair enough, he's poor old mum had passed away, but that didn't explain his performance in the first half of the year did it?

'Look on the bright side.' Alan said finally.

'Go on then, shock me.' Will sighed.

'If you hadn't been suss to the market you might have been out on your ear.'

'Says who?'

'No one; but you know what Clive's like.'

'Fuck Clive!'

'I know, I know... I'm just saying, you know what he's like.'

'I really couldn't give a fuck what he's like Al,' Will remonstrated 'do ya think he would have put anyone else in that position? Do you think if Ken had been caught like that he would have made him take the hit and cough up with his own dough?'

Alan looked deep into his glass.

'Who knows?' He lied.

'Oh fuck off Al.' Will moaned, grasping his empty glass and swinging it through the air in the direction of the barmaid.

'I'll get this!' Alan volunteered as he reached for his wallet.

'No, it's alright.'

'Go on!' Alan squawked. 'You can't afford it now son.'

It took a moment to register but when it did Will threw back his head and laughed, a genuine laugh.

It came as such a relief; he had imagined he might never experience careless laughter again.

Thank god for Alan. He was already putting everything into perspective.

A dreadful three days and nights that was all it was. So, he'd lost the best part of a hundred grand and was being visited by Cat-weasel's ugly brother in his dreams. So what? The dreams simply came from too much booze and a little too much stress, nothing a couple of quiet days on the desk and a stiff drink or three before bed couldn't sort out. The occasional crisis happened in their sort of business. That's why they earned the stupid money!

How dim witted of him to think Alan was going to give him an easy ride.

'Glad to see you haven't lost your sense of humour anyway.' Alan remarked.

'It's a good job innit?' Will had managed to relinquish with a smile.

The barmaid had finally shuffled her way over and stood glibly before them.

'Large whisky sweetheart.' Alan uttered.

'Ice?' She asked flatly.

'Yes please.'

The two friends watched her turn lethargically and fill another glass with ice before returning to the optics. In the ensuing silence Will decided that this was the opportune moment he'd been waiting for to move the conversation in his preferred direction.

'It didn't help this week, with all this going on, that I've been having full on, jump up out of bed, nightmares... did I tell you about my nightmares?' He asked casually as the barmaid returned with his laden glass.

'Nah.' Alan said, preoccupied with paying her.

'Jesus! Nightmares?' Will moaned by way of a start.

'Go on.' Alan said absent-mindedly as he received his change.

'Well me and Becks stayed at the Great Eastern on Friday night...' Will began eagerly.

'What the fuck for?'

'Doesn't matter.'

'Anyway, we were both absolutely wasted Al. Becks said she was sick all night; not that I remember, because I was out like a light.'

'Oh, you hero.' Alan remarked sarcastically.

'Yeah, I know, anyway... don't get me wrong, really nice place... probably costs a million pound a night, although I haven't had my statement yet... anyway, half way through the night I had this absolutely mad nightmare.'

Will waited until Alan had sipped his beer again, hoping for a response that didn't come.

'Yeah, anyway,' he continued 'although it wasn't exactly a nightmare; more of a vision.'

'A vision?'

'Yeah, that's what the bloke in the vision said.'

'Bloke?'

'Yes,' Will enthused. 'It was a crusty old bloke with a face as white as a ghost except he had all of these cuts around his neck. All congealed like jelly. He was hovering right above me, inches away from me face Al and his eyes were literally bulging out of his head.'

Alan nodded enthusiastically, but hoped it wasn't going to be a long story.

'And then he started ranting and I think that's what finally freaked me out.'

'Go on.' Alan said wearily.

'*I see you!*' He was shouting. '*I have found you!*' Then he was saying '*Are you our saviour? ...Pray be our saviour!*'

Will was suddenly aware of how loud and animated he'd become by the curious glance the barmaid had just given him from the other end of the bar.

'Oops,' He sighed. 'Got a bit carried away then.'

Both men lifted their glasses and drank. Alan a single gulp and Will the entire liquid content of his glass.

Alan flicked a critical eye at his friend.

'You're going to get hammered all over again then?' He asked.

'No, no,' Will said, 'I'm going to stop the moment I feel human again.'

Alan smiled now. 'The poor old boy in your vision,' he said, 'having you as his saviour... hasn't got a lot of hope has he?'

Will was busy lighting a cigarette but felt spurred onward with the last remark and launched himself into the contents of the next two night's visions.

Alan held up the palms of his hands as a buffer.

'Please Will,' he asserted, 'no more, or I'll tell you one of my sex dreams.'

Will had to concede.

He had hoped to talk the subject through to some kind of conclusion, but he knew now that he wouldn't be able to properly describe the visions to Alan or anyone else, or make them able to understand how extraordinarily real the visions were. He could picture the old man right now. Thomas. See, he'd even given him a name. Such a slight old man in a loose white shirt or gown or whatever it was; stains all over it. His hair or whatever remained of it, long and almost white and matted to his head like it hadn't seen soap or water for years.

What about his eyes? Those repulsive bulbous eyes that could only be held in by the deep furrows that surrounded them, branching out to his pointed nose and the corners of his dark mouth.

If only other people could see him just for a second, but they couldn't and they never would, so why even try? It was just a waste of time.

If it sounded completely ridiculous to himself when he tried to describe out loud anything at all about this crazy old bastard what chance was there?

Oh well, Will succumbed, while he caught the barmaid's eye again, let's just stupefy it all and anyway, perhaps Alan dismissing it had started to put the whole silly thing into perspective.

Everyone was unnerved by dreams every now and then which probably felt just as real to them as to him. He might even forget all about them in a day or two? Who knew? Although all said and done, he wasn't looking forward to bedtime.

Chapter 9 – The third visitation

I greet you again but now I am in much distress!

My clerk whose good nature I have come much to depend on hath paid me a visit with dreadful news that doth concern my wellbeing which I fear will be my final undoing.

I have thus far been made to reside in this place of bedlam. My warnings of the events I alone hath witnessed hath made a mockery of me and lead me here among the poor wretches tormented with such terrible humours that no surgeon's knife hath yet to cure.

It be a constant noise upon my ears both day and night, there being no end to those poor souls' misery, yet I am left be to practice the craft of transportation unfettered and from that hath found you.

Yet now my clerk doth speak of the counsel attended by himself where the Alderman at Southwark and the eldest brother of my dear wife do conspire to have me moved to the Marchansea gaol where all those who do violate this lands religion be kept.

Thus, I shall be caged with the worst Quakers swelling each corner with foolish piety and left to their own doing with not so much as a flock bed for comfort.

I do not follow religion sir, I have no need of it and so the charge against me will be of a pagan conspirator hard at the task to cause civil unrest.

The practice I use to seek you needs my own judged asphyxiation to calm all vibration and thus release my soul into the plain of this universe, an impossible task in the company of either gaoler or fellow prisoner.

I need then now with the utmost urgency to continue my discourse of what more I have come to witness and you must pray listen well.

The winged carriages that did cause such dreadful devastation were somehow repelled me thinks perhaps by a treaty that have led to compromise it having happened so sudden.

I have seen the mosques reach through the London skyline and wonder then what part the Moors have played to broker peace and do they now afford a greater say upon the long disputes we share with the Portuguese and the Spanish?

It has been the learning from these races of men both the Moor who did teach me it and the Portuguese gentleman that did make the introduction that I have been lessoned to leave my soul free to fly.

There is much I remain most unsure of but I must use wit in place of certainty.

I have once seen these winged carriages not only in flight but perched upon the ground in fields about Woolwich and did also watch them running at great speed to take flight with not one flap of wings.

My humble intellect can only wonder that all beasts must hath nourishment to function and though these birds be but machinery they must surely be fed by some method?

Think then sir if you will of the source, who would it be that doth the victuals for the sustenance of these rare creatures?

If it be by alchemy then I wonder if it can be of the Moors doing? This may then answer how tolerated they have become on our shores and in our great city.

Yet whoever it may be must be persuaded by reason or force to surrender their stake to the commonwealth of England for it is these birds who shall bring the destruction of London.

Please be brave dear fellow and seek counsel in haste of those who have authority, be it king or parliament, to bring about the acquisition of the source.

I wish you great fortune to find less blinkered men to hark upon than I have encountered but to action sir you must!

It had stopped raining by the time the bus had reached James's stop.

Almost proved his point he thought, as he turned the corner towards home.

James was beginning to believe that a little slice of luck was finally beginning to go his way, which was about time too as far as he was concerned.

The works had been closed for almost two weeks now and he'd thought he'd be somewhat glum when it happened, but not a bit of it, hadn't missed the place at all.

He was loath to admit it, just in case it broke the spell, but the last two weeks had actually been quite marvellous. Almost felt like a holiday, although he hadn't gone anywhere of course. It was just nice knowing that he could do if he wanted to.

That's what came of having the best part of five thousand pounds in the bank; the redundancy money.

What a clot he'd been not to have realised that redundancy pay was tax free. Well it wasn't the sort of thing he'd had to think about before, having spent so many years in state teaching. Been very lucky up to now regarding employment and his ignorance on such matters as severity payments had given him a lovely surprise when he'd read his final wage slip. Not a bean for the greedy taxman.

Debbie hadn't as yet stretched her claws out either which was perhaps a bigger shock than the wage slip. She'd just taken her usual monthly sum and left him to it. Perhaps she hadn't had a bank statement yet or perhaps she'd decided to be reasonable for a change? Either way James had resolved to keep his fingers crossed and enjoy the moment come what may.

There'd been a few complications with the teaching application but he was pretty sure that would be resolved sooner rather than later. The young lady dealing with the application had expressed a few minor concerns at the interview, but as his employment officer had very kindly pointed out, these people had to throw up a few obstacles along the way otherwise how could they justify their own existence? Everyone knows they're crying out for teachers she'd said, which seemed to be the general consensus if you followed such debates, so even James allowed himself some guarded optimism.

The timing of his application couldn't have been much better either after so much deliberation. If he'd absconded before news of the factory closure he would have completely missed out on the redundancy.

So, there it was. Nothing left to do in the meantime but wait for the correspondence and enjoy the free time, which he was in a position to do again now there was something between the lining of his wallet.

Without doubt he would have to be a little less extravagant with the money than he'd been of late if it was going to stretch anywhere; but he could forgive himself this brief break from thriftiness. He had after all been through some pretty lean times over the preceding months so he'd given himself the right to celebrate in the short term.

His birthday had been on Monday and he'd taken the boys up to the Science Museum on the Saturday before. Let then choose something each in the gift shop afterwards, barely thinking about the prices which in itself had felt wonderful and it had also been a very refreshing change to take them off to a Pizza Hut afterwards rather than one of those awful burger places.

Even the birthday itself had come and gone without being too grim. Not that there was a great deal to celebrate with becoming fifty-three whatever the circumstances he thought.

Had kept the boys' cards to open on the day; Three altogether. One from a shop which Debbie had been good enough to stump up for, signed by both boys and then a handmade card from each of them.

His gift to himself had been to find a real pub for a change where he'd spoilt himself by having some half decent pub grub.

It had even been a pleasure to pay one pound ninety-five for a pint of beer just to have someone who looked over the legal drinking age serving it.

How refreshing to feel almost normal again.

James could almost see himself sliding toward contentment. Oh, the dizzy heights to which life could once more reach!

With this lighter frame of mind James had even found himself feeling genuinely cordial towards the other inmates of his building. It was even fair to say he'd actually become quite friendly with his neighbour across the hall: the not so flying Scotsman whose name he'd found to be Brian.

He'd decided he'd been a little too quick with his accusations of idleness because Brian really did leave the place every now and then and he really was as he'd said: A pole driver. Seemed to know his stuff actually and explained the intricacies of the mechanism very aptly. Very skilled job by all accounts and can earn a fortune doing it, although there is only so much of that kind of work, hence why he always seems to be at home and whatever he does earn has to be eked out until the next job.

Had quite a bit in common really the two of them, when they chatted, although James didn't really like to dwell too much on such a depressing realisation. But they were both of a similar age. Both separated. Both stripped of house and home by their partners and deprived of any real time with their children. Although Brian's children were grown up now and only the youngest girl still lived with the mother.

Their greatest similarity however, which was a real source of pleasure for James, was their fascination with anything mechanical or indeed any clever feat of engineering.

They could talk about cars and their engines for hours, as they often did of late and were both keen to let the other share their own appreciation of anything they had recently read about or perhaps seen on the television. Brian was a bit of a formula one buff and the pair of them shared the odd heated debate as to the superiority of craftsmanship between the British constructors and their counterparts over in Italy.

Brian of course sided with the Latin corner, never wanting to give anything remotely connected to England its deserved credit. All good fun though.

James found his own enthusiasm had really quite surged since he had someone to share such interests with. Heaven knew what he'd be like when he was back in front of a classroom full of children raring for knowledge.

He'd given the library a more thorough examination and had come across one or two missed gems. He was even pondering buying a few books himself. Who knew, if he was lucky, he might even be able to pick up some of his own from the charity shops Debbie had given them to. They wouldn't be of interest to a great many he shouldn't have thought.

That could wait for now though, as James was eager to catch up on the latest teaching practises and there were numerous books printed in conjunction with the various education authorities to plough through.

He had the 'NVQ book of the Fundamentals of Engineering, Electrical and Engineering Principles' issued by BTEC and a rather generalised 'Introduction to engineering Mechanics for undergraduates.' There was certainly an abundance of publications for study purposes to choose from in the library. Most of the books were brand new as well, which was exceptional for that particular library.

Plenty then to keep him occupied until his placement came through and he knew for sure which curriculum he would be bowing to in his humble obedience.

James searched his pocket and found the metal ring holding the two Yale keys. He placed the front door key in the lock and turned slowly, then with a calculated burst of speed, threw out his free hand and grabbed the door before it had the chance to swing backward and hit the wall behind.

James still couldn't understand why it did that, although he'd spent an awful lot of time contemplating the mechanism. Every time the door had cluttered violently against the wall, in fact, while he lay with tenterhooks in his bed having heard a turn of the lock.

The hallway smelled its own peculiar smell as always, but tonight it didn't seem at all oppressive.

The second key opened the door to his room and he flicked on the light before confronting himself in the mirror.

James was happy with what he saw; a man laden with shopping and not just provisions. A few luxury items as well. Made a nice change and the library books heavy in his trusty holdall; Important books for his career. He saw a man with purpose again and would have smiled at himself if the notion hadn't have struck him as odd.

Then it suddenly occurred to him that he'd no idea of the time. An inspection of his watch revealed a quarter to seven. He'd unpack the shopping and nip over to Brian. He had the book he wanted to show him and the other thing.

Second thoughts, he'd better eat first. Sometimes popping in on Brian could end up taking all night and James was pretty sure this would be one of those nights.

He pulled the bottle out of the carrier bag and handled it with satisfaction.
A gift for Brian: It was only the supermarket brand but it was single malt. Brian would like that.

James had felt the compunction to buy it if nothing else but to allay the guilt of not inviting him out on Monday for a pint on his birthday.

Had there been anything ominous in his thoughts for not asking him to come? Was there a line he didn't want to cross in regard to their friendship? Ashamedly, James knew the answer. He knew he wanted to keep whatever relationship they shared bound tightly to his present circumstance. When he finally walked out of this dreadful place, he'd want to leave everything about it behind, everything. He knew that he'd want to reflect on his time spent here as a distant memory and completely close the chapter. He couldn't pretend that he wasn't needy of Brian's companionship, but that was all; A need of companionship so hence the whisky, a little something to dispel the guilt.

He took the other items from the bag now; the usual things. The bananas, the toilet roll and now came other things too, real treats. Biscuits as always, but ah, yes, not just the usual Rich Tea, but chocolate Digestives as well. Next was a marvellous looking pasta salad from the delicatessen counter. Not much, but enough certainly, judging by the price; finally, and quite wonderfully, a lovely round slice of goats' cheese that he just couldn't wait to bite into.

It was as good as he'd hoped, better in fact, very creamy and fresh. He could almost envisage the bracken blowing through the Welsh hills.

Having finished his meal and parcelled up the rubbish inside the carrier bag James slipped out of his room excitedly, leaving the light burning behind him. It would be wrong to take Brian's hospitality for granted, so he liked to leave the light on, just to save them both the embarrassment should it not be convenient for Brian at any time, which seemed increasingly unlikely the more he got to know the fellow. Even so, with such an event, James could simply utter 'Not to worry, wasn't stopping,' or some such phrase, then he could nip across the hall double quick and have his own door open and the light flooding out as proof of his supposed intentions.

However, this evening he needn't have had such concern as just as soon as he'd knocked, he could hear his friend clear his throat as he approached the door.

'Be wi'ya in a sec.' Came the thick Glaswegian brogue. Now James could hear the safety chain being pulled across and the low rasps from Brian's chest before the door was edged open.

'Oh, it's the Dean.' Brian mumbled under his thick greying moustache before pushing the door too, then releasing it with another rattle of the chain.

'Welcome ye, welcome all.' Came the greeting as Brian stepped back into the room and waved his visitor inside.

'Good evening to you too dear sir.' James answered in the same spirit as he entered the room shielding the contents of his hands behind his back.

'I come bearing gifts and enlightenment.'
Brian's room was a good deal larger than his own, which was fair enough as far as James was concerned, considering the time the poor chap had existed in this awful place. It had still come as a bit of a shock to discover his own room had been Brian's first billet. It was

quite an accomplishment to persuade the landlords to move him when he thought of the dealings he'd had with them himself and he was happier to dwell on that aspect of the move rather than imagine Brian and all of his habits let loose on the same mattress he now called his own. Such thoughts always made him wince slightly as he perched himself down carefully on the edge of Brian's grubby quilt but whatever the state of the room it did always make sense for the pair of them to spend their time in here rather than in his own room.

The furniture was virtually identical but it had found a much better perspective here and apart from anything else it was nice to leave the smoke behind when he went back across the hall.

Brian, as hoped, was overjoyed with his gift and as anticipated was quite insistent that they both sample the goods immediately.

Thankfully his friend had a favourite tumbler, so although you could never by any stretch of the imagination call any of his humble collection of glassware clean, you could at least be sure you weren't receiving a receptacle that included something fresh from his brown lips lurking there in wait on the rim.

The whiskey itself was very nice. Much smoother than the stuff Brian normally had to offer, but then again what with the amount he went through it was unlikely he could afford much else but the cheapest blends.

James watched his friend take a long slow draw from his tumbler then smack his sticky lips together in loud appreciation.

'There's ya true dram.' He declared, holding up the remainder of the golden liquid to the bare bulb on the ceiling and setting to work the light amber tanning through the elegant crystal.

'Mmm,' James agreed, 'good stuff.'
'Aye.'

The two men sat facing each other in silent appreciation of their drinks but once James had emptied his glass, he set it down excitedly on the dust clad carpet and turned his attention to the book he had carefully propped face down on the bed so as not to give away the content.

'Now I've softened you up a bit, I think it's time to go on the offensive.'

Brian looked at him ruefully as James patted the book that was still lying there before him obscured in the crumpled quilt.

'I have sir, within this book a short paragraph which will, I hope, align your misguidance as to the true master of Formula racing.'

Brian countered with a derisive yawn before he spoke.

'Don't worry, I've spied ya book and am ready for ye and believe me, whatever it is you've got between those pages, I shan't be changing ma mind as to whom the master is.'

'No, no, no, wouldn't expect anything else from a Fangio fan.' James retorted, as he opened the back pages at the appendix and quickly ran his finger downwards in search of the required section.

'Just wanted to settle that little dispute we were having about your Mr. Fangio and my Mr. Moss.'

'Ya better have another drop now then,' Brian said as he stooped heavily on one knee with the bottle and filled James's glass almost half way, 'before I cast ya out.'

It was all James could do to lift his head from the pillow come morning.

The sun was streaming in from the crack in the curtains, lighting up his bed and near blinding him in the one eye that seemed willing to function. God only knew what time it was but it certainly felt late.

Hadn't even heard the Bosnian exodus down the stairs this morning, or the crashing as the front door hit the wall repeatedly on their way out. Thank god for that, he considered. Wasn't sure his brain could take that sort of trauma today.

Didn't actually ever want to move again but he could feel something rising upwards from his stomach which meant he'd have to at least sit up long enough for whatever it was to pass through his mouth. Thankfully it was nothing more than wind.

There was a decision to make now when he most wanted decisions deferred, but here it was, did he do something sensible for once and use the rest of his strength to clamber down the hall to consume vast quantities of water which might help alleviate some of the torture the vast quantities of whisky had inflicted on him or did he simply fall back on the bed and hope he'd survive without it?

How on earth did they manage to drink the whole bottle of good stuff and the best part of Brian's usual poison? He pondered while gazing up at the ceiling cracks after he'd made his choice.

Oh, but Brian's expression when he'd read the paragraph that explained Moss had beaten Fangio at Aintree in fifty-five, in the only race they'd started on a level playing field as team mates with Mercedes. It was absolutely priceless that expression.

James found himself chuckling despite the affect it was having on his head.

Last night had really been fun. It had almost felt like happiness.

Becky pressed the dimmer switch and very quickly adjusted the strength of the lights that had just sent a sharp pain through her squinting eyes.

She was just shattered now but Will was in bed on his back and snoring for England. It was funny how he could always get back to sleep even after screaming the house down she reflected with some irritation.

She slumped heavily onto the smaller settee.

'Shit! What was that!' She gasped.

Something had just dug into a buttock so hard she had felt it hit a bone.

'Jesus.' She groaned.

Of course, it was one of Will's books that he always left strewn around the apartment. Had to be didn't it? The arguments they'd had about those bloody books.

He'd pile them up in every room if she let him and the amount of toes the pair of them had stubbed on those bloody books; But then the sudden image of seeing Will hopping around clutching a foot made Becky giggle for a moment despite her exhaustion, though she soon decided she was far too tired for any sort of prolonged merriment. Even a slight giggle had been enough to make her neck creek and her head ache. If she was going to waste any more energy and feel the pain from it she would use it on something far more worthwhile like crying. God! She could use a good cry now if it wasn't so bloody tiring.

It did it to her this lack of sleep. It actually sort of sent her a bit mental; Mental like her idiot snoring husband.

Now all of a sudden she really was crying. Silently, or as near as she could keep it as the tears snaked their way down her taut cheeks and along her nose and onto her top lip.

Becky lifted her lower lip to meet them and tasted the salt. She didn't want to start calling him those sorts of names, that silly man lying in her bed finally asleep, bless him.

She was ashamed now for calling him mental and even for being pissed off with him at all. He'd only just lost his mum a few months ago and it was such a short time a few months, she really did have to try and remember that. She always had to think what she'd be like if she lost her mum. No, actually she didn't, couldn't really. It was unthinkable to be honest so she just had to realise how screwed up it made you. For a long while, well, forever really. They said some people never truly recover. She knew that's what she'd be like.

Will was falling on his arse at work too, or so it would seem without him saying too much. It was what he didn't say. He used to get home from work and he was either talking shop which she couldn't always follow, or he was talking dull office politics which was much like listening to a broken record.

But it was his face in the morning as he kissed her goodbye that really told her there was something up.

She loved him so much that man who stopped her from sleeping. Even though he spent half of his own sleeping time farting and making other peculiar noises, even though his well-being was just a constant worry for her now. Even though his drinking and his arrogance drove her to despair sometimes there was so much more about him. She knew that, course she did.

There were his silly books for a start. She said she hated them but she didn't. They were one of the things that made him... well, him.

Becky searched limply around with a hand and found the book that had injured her. She picked it up awkwardly and twisted it around to look at the cover. Such a heavy bloody thing she couldn't keep her grip and watched it fall back onto the sofa.
There was something ugly on the cover, perhaps a human figure but really no more than a blob if anything. The writing too seemed impossible to decipher, just a whole lot of swirling letters scratched across the blob thing that faded in and out with different thicknesses and colour.

Becky squinted to read something she'd just seen at the bottom of the cover, small lettering but much plainer.

Heaven sake! She thought with disgust once she'd read it, how could she not have guessed? A book of dreams written by someone unpronounceable; it had to be though didn't it? Will had already started to obsess about those silly nightmares of his and now he'd started reading about them as well, just so he could obsess some more.

If this was the first one, he'd bought you could bet he'd have another dozen before long and then another dozen about ghosts and wot not.

He was always doing that. If he found a book he liked he'd go out and get everything the author had ever written. All in one go.

The worst time was when he started buying art books. There was never one that fit the book shelves. The bloody things were propped up everywhere until she lost it with him one day.

Becky sighed deeply and miserably at the inevitability of it all. The third bedroom was a virtual library now with book cases all around the room.

Becky had to admit it looked quite nice when it was tidy, which was only when she'd tidy it but what she really found annoying was out of all of his books there wasn't really anything she would want to read. There wasn't an enormous amount of novels in there and the few there were seemed mostly old fashioned and by dead authors. In fact, most of the books were non-fiction so it felt like a glorified reference library; shelf upon shelf of amazingly tedious facts, figures, dates and analysis; fact upon, fact upon very dull fact.

'You're right,' Will would say whenever she chose to have a snipe about them, 'but that's why I'm such a clever bastard.'

It was true as well, Will was a clever bastard and no doubt the books had helped make him so. He loved his books and had done since he was a little boy and the proof was there on the shelves because he had kept so many of them. The history books, various editions of the Guinness book of records, Encyclopaedias for children and there was still nothing he liked more than to sink his teeth into a huge volume or two or a pictorial about the art of photography while he was getting smashed.

Will was snoring more than ever now, the noise vibrating around the whole apartment.

Becky knew she wouldn't get anymore sleep but she wasn't annoyed anymore. She couldn't be when she thought about him as a solemn little boy sitting alone in his room reading books.

'I don't like talking to Australians normally you know... and I know you don't wanna talk to me... but if you did, just say you did, you'd be banging on about Australia; how far you'd be prepared to drive to a restaurant. How it's always fucking hot, s'cuse my French, and you don't even need a proper coat and all that stuff about how much you like England and the pubs and all that, so on and so on.'

She was gone then, over to the other end of the bar to serve someone else and quite pleased she looked too for the chance to get away.

She was obviously a very nice girl. Far too polite to stay where she was once she'd finished serving and was reluctantly back opposite him sipping on her coke.

Will wondered how used to wearing a blouse she was. She looked more of a jeans and tee shirt kind of girl. Last thing she wanted was a suit chatting her up. He hoped she didn't really think he was trying to pull her.

'Hello again.' He said.

He drunk a good draft of lager and suppressed a burp.

'Sorry.' He mumbled and she smiled her meek acceptance.

'You know I'm not trying to chat you up though dont'cha? I only got married a couple of months ago.'

She kept her smile in place.

'Thank god for my wife.' He mumbled as the girl escaped again.

Will finished his drink and slipped out onto the street.

It was still so warm outside and the sky was dark and blue. The black cabs flew by in glowing yellow reflections.

He really didn't want to go home to dream.

Company would have been nice now. Becks ideally, but the guys who he'd been to dinner with would have done.

The clients they had taken out seemed like they would have been fine as well on the face of it.

It was them that had requested somewhere they could have cocktails and found it a fun idea to be taken to the Ice Tea Bar. They seemed properly up for any sort of craic when Al was telling them some of those infamous stories of his. They were sinking enough of the silly drinks as well, all with enough measures of vodka and whatever so you could properly feel it, so Will was sure in his mind that a walk around the corner would also have been thought of as fun for them after the Ice Tea. If nothing else they were Norwegians for Christ's sakes, weren't they meant to party through instinct? and what with Stringfellow's just a stone's throw away?

It was a real surprise and not to say a disappointment that there wasn't a single taker to move on.

It had all hinged on Al of course. If he wanted to go on, he would have had everyone up for it. That's what Al could do when he wanted to, but tonight he didn't.

He'd turned into Captain Sensible of late bless him.

'Not on a school night.' He'd said before explaining the phrase to his new Viking friends who had laughed and held their heads to convey a mock hangover.

That gave Peta the chance to baulk, miserable fucker that he was and the Vikings had quickly regained their professional conscientiousness and had no doubt opted to get secretly pissed in their hotel bar once they'd said their goodbyes.

Well fuck em! Will thought. He was going to have his night out regardless.

There were a couple more boozers in sight as he looked down St Martin's Lane toward the Opera House but if they were as drab as the one he'd just walked out of he could cut across to Leicester Square and maybe up to Soho.

He quite fancied something a bit swanky, a bit of music, a million pounds for a bottle of trendy lager.

He'd have to call Becks and tell her he was still with the clients', she'd be fine with that.

Sometime later he found himself in another pub even drabber than the first one. Wooden panels partitioning areas of the bar. It seemed almost full of strangers, all strangers to one another.

There was an enormous man with scraggly hair and an unkempt beard who was wearing round and frameless glasses, standing alone at the bar. He was staring blankly at himself in the cloudy mirror behind the optics.

'You look like a professor.' Will observed nudging him gently. 'Are you a professor?'

'Afraid not.' The man replied in a clipped tone without averting his eyes.

'That's a shame!' Will continued undeterred. 'I could really use the advice of a professor right now.'

He had to stop just then and close his eyes to think of what advice it was he needed. He was so fucking drunk... drunk and tired.

'Oh, what d'ya know about Astral projection?' He blurted having suddenly remembered.

'I think someone's astrally projecting to me you see?' He explained. 'If that's what you call it?'...visions anyway... lots of ranting.'

Fuck, that'll scare him off, Will thought, but the man didn't move away or move at all other than to part his lips, not that Will could see them move under all of that beard.

'It's all to do with density.' The man sighed. 'If you're able to lower your vibrational frequency to a low enough level you can supposedly shed your physical shell.'

'Wow!' Will enthused. 'You really are a scientist!'

'No, I'm not.' Came the next clipped response.

'But can you travel to the future then?'

'Some have claimed they are able to traverse time, yes...'

'Fucking hell!' Will exulted, 'I knew it! It's fucking brilliant!'

'If it's to be believed.' The bearded man sneered,

'I believe it!' Will said. 'I really believe it now! ...look, can I buy you a drink?' Will offered, staggering backward with his hand in his trouser pocket searching for his cash.

'No thank you.'

'Really?'

'Yes.'

'But you've really helped me a lot.' Will said, clinging to the man's arm to steady himself.

'Please!' the large man exerted himself, pushing Will away before turning to face him for the first time.

'Sorry.' Will said genuinely. 'You've just been very, really very, very helpful and clever and that, so I just wanted to buy you a drink.'

'Just! leave me alone.' The man replied.

Will winced intuitively, unable to actually feel the embarrassment.

'I'm going to go.' He said meekly pulling himself upright. 'Sorry.' He said again.

He closed his eyes once more to recall something relevant he needed to remember ...and that was it he thought, he just had to remember he was going to leave.

He switched once more to the man with the beard who had returned to stare at his own reflection somewhere behind the bar.

Will couldn't resist one last question although he knew it was going to exacerbate. He stepped up to the man and tapped gently on an elbow.

'Just tell me,' he said, 'if you're like... *not* a scientist, how do you know all of that stuff?'

'I'm educated.' Came the immediate and blunt response.

I liked that, Will thought, as he staggered his way out into the busy night. I'll have to remember that one.

It was only a short while later that he began reflecting on his meeting with the bearded man.

What a wanker! Will decided, looking at his own reflection in a mirror. Who the fuck stares at themselves all night in a mirror?

He'd finally found his swanky bar.

There was a Brandy Alexander on order. Fucking lovely! Brandy and cream though, wasn't quite sure how that was going to stay down.

Anyway, fucking educated! Cheeky bastard! Scruffy bastard who probably didn't have no friends. Sure-fire virgin you could bet your life. Habitual masturbator, Will was sure he'd be the type wanking over small boys and male ballet dancers.

The barmaid who he had barely noticed when he'd placed his order came and placed his drink before him. Beautiful if you like that sort of thing he thought. Chiselled cheeks, pulled back hair and lipstick like blood. Like one of them guitarists from a Robert Palmer video.

'Fuck, that don't look like what I was expecting.' He grumbled.

'Shame.' The girl replied. 'Five pounds seventy-five.'

The drink tasted as bad as it looked and Will suddenly had the urge to throw it back across the bar but he resisted. He'd have one of them Mexican beers next time.

At least there was some really good dance music being played. Not that he'd be in a fit enough state to dance unless he slowed down the drinking.

Once he got his beer, he could maybe fight his way through the crowd and get himself into the space over by the far wall and take it easy for a bit.

He was looking forward to being played with by the bunch of beauties who were dancing together near there. One of them would collar him when they saw he was alone. He could show her and all her friends his wedding ring then. Just got married to my best mate Becks he'd say.

Fuck! Now he remembered, he hadn't phoned her like he was meant to and it was too late now, wake her up and she might want him to come home.

He wanted her to come to him really and wondered what time the place shut. She could have a quick shower and get dressed and that and jump in a cab. He could meet her outside and pay the fare and they could go to the Empire in Leicester Square. Do some dancing; he wouldn't be wobbly by then. They could have some proper cocktails.

She wouldn't come though would she? No, not if he thought about it properly. Will was suddenly despondent. It was too late really and if he did ask her or even phone her at all she would make him go home. School night and all that.

He could've cried really. He could have easily cried.

'Mind!' Someone yelled once he'd finally bought his beer and was fighting his way through the crowd.

'Move your fucking fag!' A girl shouted again before stooping to inspect the hem of her dress in the half light.

'Sorry!' He called back.

Will found an empty space and bit on the slice of lime that had been pushed into the spout of his bottle.

The beer had been drunk before he had even stubbed his cigarette out on the carpet. He'd have to fight his way back now. He'd get two bottles next time he decided and he would have a large scotch and just down it quickly at the bar so he didn't need to carry it.

'Fucking hell, Becks... where are ya mate? He mumbled to his reflection as he stood again waiting to be served.

'I wish you were here.'

****

What have you got to say for yourself tonight then Thom? He asked a bright light that had caught the blur of indistinct shapes which were just out of reach from where he found himself, stranded as he was on the cobbled forecourt of Charing Cross station.

He had an ache on his knee where he had fallen and when he pushed his finger through the hole that had been made in his trousers, he could feel the sting and sense the blood slowly oozing out.

There were no more cigarettes.

He was undone... wasn't that the phrase Thom had sometimes used?

It was dark, really dark and quiet and then suddenly it was light and he awoke in his suit on one of the sofas in the apartment.

'Veronica darling, are you going to be long?'

'Veronica?'

She stepped out of the door and showed her slightly perplexed
face. Her lips surprisingly blazon with red lipstick.

'Hello darling,' she snapped, 'getting up?'

'No, just need to go.'

'Oh,' she said, 'thought you'd been'

'No darling.' He said with a yawn.

She patted him softly on the shoulder as she brushed her way
past clear of him.

'You're very smart.' He complimented.

'Oh well... you know how these bloody councillors are.'

James smiled sympathetically.

'You smell rather nice too.' He said rubbing his eyes.

'I just hope it works.' She sighed.

That was one of the wonderful things about Veronica; she'd take
on anyone and anything that confronted itself in pursuit of the
better good, especially if she was trying to achieve something that
would benefit her children. So naturally shy and timid but she'd rise
to any challenge.

'Well I've really got to go now then darling!' He called.

'Fine!' She answered from their bedroom. 'Go then darling!' She
encouraged as she inspected herself in the mirror one last time.

James stood over the bowl but no matter how hard the effort or
desire he remained frustrated.

'I shall miss you today!' He shouted from over his shoulder.

'Oh, I'll be back for lunch!' She called.

'Mmm.' James mused, thinking of what he might prepare for
her return.

'Right, I'll be off then.' She whispered, having sneaked up on him.

'Oh Veronica!'

'Oops... so sorry darling... you haven't sloshed have you?'

'No.' He said recovering from his fright.

'Tu-dah-loo then.' She said breathing coffee and lipstick into his neck.

****

James tossed himself over.

He was awake now and he really did have to pee. Thank heavens he was never tricked into it by his dreams.

He'd get up in a minute and slip his trousers on and just hope the bathroom was empty.

He'd been dreaming about his first wife an awful lot lately. Not that there had ever been a time when he'd completely managed to stop thinking about her if he was honest. He'd certainly tried. It didn't seem fair on Deborah... a sort of betrayal somehow.

He couldn't prevent the dreams of course but he had always made a point never to ponder them while awake. Now, however, it didn't matter and he had all the time in the world to spend pondering; here alone on his bed again in the middle of the morning.

He just wondered how Veronica would react if she knew the sort of existence he'd allowed himself to be coerced into.

Would she be pleased? Would she gloat?
Somehow, he doubted it. She was never one to be vindictive, not even after the unforgivable way he'd treated her. She'd probably feel disappointment for him being the woman she was.

Oh, but what about the woman she became? James could finally indulge in that question to his heart's content and the realisation of that was just the lift he needed to make the effort to rise up and get decent to try his luck in the loo and thankfully it was unoccupied.

He sat in near darkness and remained there for a while with his thoughts.
Did she ever remarry? He certainly hoped so, Veronica deserved happiness.

Of course, the big question that had always needed addressing in his mind that he had conveniently managed to avoid for so very long was there before him now, waiting, patience expired. Had she ever adopted?

She and James had talked about it long enough. She did so want children of her own. She was set on it really.

James was never averse to the idea and he had certainly made all the right noises to suggest that when Veronica decided the time was right, he would be in unison with her.

It made using her infertility as an excuse to leave her all the more despicable. Totally inexcusable and to think that at the time he chose that reason because he knew it would bring him a little sympathy and support from their families and friends. It worked in some quarters. His mother had been in his corner from the moment he had told her, not he felt from a mothers' loyalty, but more the instinctive pang of a maternal grandmother.

What a coward he had been, yet even now he wondered if he would have had the courage to make a more honest job of it. What else was there for him to say? That he had become bored with his ordinary life? That his extraordinary wife had made him feel average? Those things yes, those things for sure, but there was really only one emotion that drove everything, lust, pure and simple.

Of course, he was being relentlessly pushed to leave Veronica by this young, fresh, uncomplicated woman who had up to that point been the willing recipient of every sexual advance he had made toward her and at any given time.

James could hardly call Deborah any of those things now, perhaps young, relatively speaking. She certainly wasn't uncomplicated, which should however, he decided, never be mistaken for sophisticated.

They never had a great deal in common he and Deborah after the first flourish of their relationship, which in essence had only ever been based on sex. He still couldn't decide if he had discovered that in hindsight or if his subconscious had conveniently brushed the notion aside.

Fucked like a banshee did Debbie and was quite insatiable for a while.

The irony still stung a little to think she chose sex as the issue to finally pack his bags.

Sex was never an issue with Veronica. She was never one to get bogged down with the domestic or personal. To be honest it didn't register on her radar as necessary. She did it of course if she was asked to but it was of little importance to her.

She was the sort of person who had very much wanted to change the world and she had the tenacity to really try and do it. Education mainly; a fight from within as it were. She was already making her mark within the N.U.T. all that time ago when he knew her.

He could quite easily see her on the Board of Education if she was still at it, although it was quite difficult to notice what her achievements had been if that were the case, however ungracious that sounded.

You only had to look at the school his boys attended as an example.

The headmistress herself had very little competence when it came to grammar if the letters the boys brought home were anything to go by and the teachers seemed to come and go from one year to the next. No continuity which was thought to be of such great importance when he first taught.

He was very much looking forward to discovering the current government directives and the way the people on the front line had adapted them to make them at all practical. He was sure that method of working would still be as necessary now as ever.

Hopefully he really would be finding all of this out first hand in the not too distant future.

Who knew? Perhaps Veronica had decided to stay on the front line? A part of James liked to think she did in all honesty. She was so very good at it and so amazingly dedicated too. It was awful to think she may have been propelled so far upward that she no longer had regular interaction with the children. That for her had been what mattered essentially, the education of children, although of course one couldn't dismiss the thought that if she had followed the usual career path, she would by now have become at least a headmistress. Frontline enough he supposed; no doubt sending her children home with perfectly concise and grammatically correct information.

The conjecture was endless.

James returned to his room and removed his trousers then lay there upon his bed absorbed in his remorse, recumbent in misery.

He would have to shake himself out of it, try to focus on the positive things.

He didn't regret the whole of his relationship with Deborah, of course not. He would never be without his boys... although, however he tried to deflect the thought... he was... in the main.

Wasn't at all at his best now, not at all, but he knew he would snap out of it. Just give the nose a bit of a wipe with his handkerchief and he'd be fine.

That was the trouble with endless contemplation and supposition; it often left you feeling terribly sad.

He spotted something just then through the watery blur. Some sort of creature lumbering its way across the ceiling toward the light socket. James thought he'd concentrate on that for a bit, a welcome distraction.

Wasn't a spider, wasn't a cockroach... thank heaven! Something with wings evidently, which it hadn't chosen to use until just then.

Lucky little thing thought James, to have a choice like that.

He knew he would have to remove whatever it was as it flittered aimlessly around the unlit bulb.

He couldn't open a window unfortunately as they were sealed up by the landlord as a security measure, so the trousers would have to go back on. Sneak the little bugger out of the front door if he could catch it.

Do you know what though? James thought suddenly, if the trousers were to go back on, perhaps they should stay on for a while? He could sneak his little roommate out of the front door then nip back into the bathroom if he could and give the face and pits a bit of a scrub.

Would be nice to feel free himself if only for a few hours.

The money wasn't holding up as well as he'd hoped... without fresh money coming in he could only look and watch what he had slowly dwindle away. But there was enough for the occasional soiree into town if he needed it. Nothing too lavish; a few pints in *Parvs* and who knew? Perhaps he'd tap on Brian's door later and have another nice little tipple with him.

'Sweetheart.' Will whispered, but she didn't stir.

'Becks.' He persisted.

She moved then. Lifted her head above the duvet and opened an eye momentarily then closed it again.

'Come on sweetheart,' Will said 'I've made you breakfast.'

Becky opened both of her eyes this time and looked up at him with an element of disdain.

Will very carefully waved the coffee cup by its saucer in her line of vision.

'That's hardly breakfast.' She mumbled thickly.

'It's your usual breakfast though isn't it?' He said unperturbed.

'It's not food.'

'Clearly Baba,' Will beamed 'but if you want a proper breakfast I shall make you a proper breakfast.'

'God's sake,' she moaned 'what's got into you?'

She pulled the duvet over her face.

'I'm just in a good mood that's all.' Will said chirpily. 'There's already a bit of sun out there. I woke up nice and fresh and early and I'm going off to work now to seek my fortune!'

'Sod off then,' Becky mumbled wearily from under the covers, 'just leave the coffee on my side.'

Will slid out of the apartment block and stepped into the sunshine with a real sense of euphoria and looked at his surroundings as if with fresh eyes.

He saw the familiar return to how it should be and how it truly was rather than the distorted wreckage his imagination had conceived; the carefully landscaped gardens surrounding the block and the young trees which lined the ornate boundary fence. He took a moment to survey the grand detached houses along the road and the comforting sight of the pub roof just over in the distance. All of this set off by the morning sun.

Will was almost giddy with jubilation. Such a contrast to the grim scene his mind had cast just yesterday and for several of the preceding weeks and now the smoking rubble and the charred remains of the devastating storm had disappeared with his hysteria.

Thank god he'd finally come to his senses and thought the whole thing out.

Will had finally realised that it was Matt's schoolbooks that had started the whole nonsense off.

It happened late the night before as he sat on the train drunk and dreading the usual assault on his senses which he knew would happen the moment he fell asleep.

He was pawing over all the details he could remember from the dreams, trying to make sense of them, hoping to decipher something of use he might have missed before. A use for what he was still unsure of but he couldn't stop going over and over everything endlessly.

What he had longed for was advice. He wanted Thom, this creation he'd brought to life, to help him escape the terror that was coming. Remove the obligations that were being thrust upon him. Let slip a get out or a safe place to hide. He might even have mentioned someone else between the frightening rhetoric who Will would recognise from the twentieth century. Someone else who he hoped Thom had been in contact with, maybe a big shot, powerful enough to take action to stop the impending doom he prophesised.

He was so fucking desperate.

Then it happened… a stray thought out of nowhere. Something tugging at his memory just as he was berating the usefulness of the reference books he had assembled.

It was the odd way Thom had of speaking that had always rang a distant bell, yet he couldn't think for the life of him where he'd come upon that sort of enunciation before. Then it suddenly occurred to him that he'd read some form of old-fashioned speech in one of Matt's school folders.

The timing of his discovery couldn't have come any sooner as far as he was concerned. The visions or nightmares or whatever he'd perceived them to be were beginning to make him deranged.

So, devoid of sleep, drunk and barely clinging to reason he made it home and was in through the front door then straight into the spare room and heaving his way through Matt's old books like a man possessed and he was right! Thank god.

He'd found it quickly; the passage he'd been hoping to find was there in black and white in his trembling hands.

'Our maid Jane called up about three in the morning, to tell us of a great fire she saw in the city. So, I rose, and slipped on my night-gown and went to her window, and thought it be on the back side of Mark Lane at the farthest; but, being unused to such fires as followed, I thought it far enough off, and so went to bed again and to sleep...
By and by Jane comes and tells me that she hears that above three hundred houses have burned down tonight by the fire we saw, and that it is now burning down all Fish street by London Bridge. So I made myself ready presently, and walked to the Tower; and there got up upon one of the higher places,... and there I did see the houses at the end of the bridge all on fire, and an infinite great fire on this and the other side... of the bridge... so down (I went), with my heart full of trouble, to the Lieutenant of the Tower, who tells me that it began this morning in the King's baker's house in Pudding-lane.'

Will could barely begin to describe his relief. Certainly not in any considered way.

He'd so wanted to wake Becks and express something for how he was feeling. He wanted to hug her and jump around the room. He would show her the quotation that had been carefully cut out and pasted onto the page above a crude yet sweet picture of London in flames drawn by his brother's own hand.

He decided against it in the end. It was really quite late and she'd smell his breath and think he was drunk; well, obviously he was drunk, so she would have gone berserk at him for disturbing her and wouldn't have listened to anything he tried to explain anyway.

Instead he poured himself a large celebratory scotch and sat down on one of the sofas with the folder.

There was only half a dozen or so pages but they were all about the Great Fire of 1666. There were pictures of noblemen and a number of quotes from eye witnesses like the one from Pepys that he had just read to himself. Will was struck to find that regardless of who had given the quote the style of wording was essentially the same.

Any one of them, or rather, each one of them could have inspired the creation of Thom in his thick skull.

It was laughingly obvious now, but then things always were in hindsight.

It would have saved him an awful lot of distress if he had realised sooner. There was always a rational explanation if you really focused on finding it. He just hadn't taken a step back and thought about it hard enough.

Will wouldn't beat himself up too much though; he had after all read through every single one of Matt's school books and even the folders at some point. But what he read didn't seem to register a lot of the time, probably as he was a little worse for wear when he did start to read them. He really hadn't spent any time, or at least paid much attention to the text books with such small writing or even the stuff Matt had merely cut out and stuck into the folders.

All he could honestly think he had remembered clearly were the date stamps on the library books and that only because they had made him ache for a moment or two, simply because they had shown the books were due back in the library just a few days after Matt had died.

Well anyway, it was obvious now that the seeds for his little spell of lunacy had slipped into his subconscious while he was off guard, simply enjoying pawing through the exercise books in Matt's scrawny handwriting and smiling at the pictures; the diluted residue of his brother.

Sometimes it had even felt as though they were sharing a conversation, or rather, it felt as if he was listening to Matt reading to him out loud like he sometimes did in the summer when it was bedtime but still light enough to read.

All the stuff about the Great Fire of course but also everything you cared to know about the process of frogspawn evolving into frogs and such like. All narrated by Matt's young voice.

Matt had got a gold star for that, probably because of the great drawing he'd done of the frogs.

He'd received a gold star for the Great Fire project too which was stuck at the bottom of the last page just under another picture of the fire, this time with plague rats running away from a city in flames.

'Good work!' The teacher had scrawled.
He'd deserved that star Will decided. It was a bloody well-presented project for someone of that age.

'Good for you bruv.' Will whispered, raising his glass upward toward the ceiling then draining the remainder of the whisky.

He went to bed then, a relieved man determined to enjoy the first peaceful slumber for what had seemed an age with happy thoughts of his big brother comforting him.

He couldn't wait to explain it to Becks and he'd even gone to bed looking forward to getting to work.

Becky called him as soon as she arrived at her office.

'Vendibles.' Will answered vibrantly.

'My god you're cheerful today!' Becky was quick to observe.

'Yes, I bloody am.' He agreed.

'Sorry I was so grumpy this morning.'

'That's alright.'

'So, what's put you in such a good mood then?'

'I think I've sorted myself out Becks.' Will announced happily.

'What do you mean?'

'I've got my head around the nightmares.'

'Right.' She answered cautiously.

'Yeah, I finally realised where I conjured that character up from.'

'Character?'

'You know, Thom!' The old bloke giving me the he bee gee bees every night! It's because I've been reading all of those bloody history books Becks... Matt's school books you see? I made him up after reading my bruv's history project and all of those diaries I bought.'

Will paused for a response but was met with a pregnant silence as Becky absorbed what he was saying.

'I know it sounds mad,' he continued 'but I think that's all it was. Didn't realise you see? I must have read a load of stuff when I was pissed.'

Still there was no response.

'Go on, say something.' He urged her.

'I don't know what to say,' was all she could manage, 'I'm just so... relieved you know?'

'Not half as relieved as me darling... I bet you thought I was going bonkers didn't you?'

'Of course not.' Becky replied.

'Well I wish I'd been so sure.' Will confessed.

'Oh Will.' Becky sighed.

'Doesn't matter, doesn't matter... it's alright now thank fuck... so anyway sweetheart,' Will said lightly, 'that's why I'm in a fantastic mood and now I can put my overzealous imagination to some practical use and try to dream up a decent trading strategy.'

'You still need to slow down you know.' Becky warned.

'I know,' Will agreed, 'and I'm going to sweetheart, I promise, it's just that I'm so over the bloody moon today!'

Once they had said their goodbyes and he had reluctantly replaced the receiver, Will sat stiffly at his desk with pen in hand poised purposely over his day book. He was very serious about focusing his thoughts on improving his work performance, even more acutely aware of the nagging concern that was always at the back of his mind of the size of the coming outlay that he would be facing, the debts, which he'd let mount up when he'd thought he could pay them off and of course the beautiful yet ridiculously expensive car he'd signed up for which would always have been a push to afford even in the best of times, yet for the moment at least the morning's euphoria made him optimistic.

Will felt he'd turned a corner. In fact, he was so upbeat that he'd even slid the Aston brochure into his hand on the way out of the apartment. It had been the first time in weeks that he'd even so much as looked at the cover, but on the train that morning, he didn't only read through the thing but actually contemplated owning the car again. Okay, hadn't a hope of affording it as things stood that was sure enough, but he'd already paid the deposit so he'd have to set about changing the situation.

Clive would, if as usual, be thinking about the bonuses in around six weeks' time so Will had until then to put in a much improved performance. Maximum effort which he and Clive both knew had been lacking for bloody ages. From now on it would have to be onwards and upwards.

The first thing he was going to do was one of his famous overviews which he'd got out of the habit of doing: through sheer laziness really. It had taken up too much of his time had been his thinking when he'd dropped it, but now he was going to make a point of finding the time. If it didn't give him any decent leads, which had often been the case in the past, it would at least serve the purpose of making Clive aware that he was making a conscious effort at improvement. That had to hold some sway when the sour old bastard begun making his calculations.

Will needed to sit down with the research boys again and have a thorough conflab on the state of the world markets. Get a little bit of useful conjecture out of them rather than just the usual system generated projections they produced for the entire trading desk.

He'd have to start inviting himself out to lunch with one or two of the more clued up brokers too. Hadn't done that in ages because it wasn't something he enjoyed doing on his own as most of them were such slimy fuckers really and it was always a bugger getting Al or Ken to go along. Still, if he had to do it on his own he would.

'The market seems quiet to me.' Alan commented an hour or so later as he ripped the packaging off of another of his mid-morning snacks. 'Why are you on overdrive?' He asked.

Will was watching the screens intently with a phone screwed to his ear.

'Just getting a few little fills.' He said engrossed. 'I reckon it's going to go up a little when NYBOT opens.'

'Okay,' Alan said, 'you 'de man.' Although he wasn't quite convinced, still it was nice to see the boy make an effort for a change.

Pray do not flinch from me and tame your discomfort for I have but a few more days and now must pass the most grievous knowledge you must be party to though I be loath to share it for I am leaving this bedlam.

I visit you in hope that you have by now begun to attend to the urgent matter I have been pressing you toward and you have found in your labour some alliance for now it would seem certain you shall be my only prolocutor.

I am vexed with such pity but I feel a duty to take this last opportunity to strengthen your purpose.

Brace yourself then for the most terrible disclosure I have been hiding thus to spare your fortitude until now… for I have seen London disappear in a single blast of light sir and though I have sought in endless transmutation to see the city later I have found nothing but a storm of soil and earth ever after.

Doomsday is in your time poor fellow. Use courage. Make haste.

'I need to turn the light on,' Becky asserted, 'mind your eyes.'

Will shut his eyes tightly then summoned them open again. 'What time is it?' He mumbled.

'Look at the clock.' She said sternly as she sat at her vanity unit and began stroking her wet hair into a decent shape with her brush.

Will looked at the clock through bleary eyes.

'Fuck.' He said and lay back down.

There was a fair chance he would have stayed there all day if Becky hadn't turned on the hairdryer. He couldn't bear it this morning, it was as if the noise was coming from inside his head. He struggled up from under the quilt and stood there motionless for a while until he had his balance.

'I'm dying.' He moaned.

Becky switched the dryer off. 'What?' She asked impatiently.

'I said I'm dying.'

Becky switched the dryer back on in disgust then switched it off again.

'You didn't have to go out again did you?' She spat from the mirror.

'Look, I've already told you it was work.' He sighed.

'They were brokers Will! Since when did you have to go out with brokers?'

Will shook his head dismally.

'I've also told you these guys give us the best fills so we have to keep them sweet.'

'Well that sounds exactly like Alan's words to me, but I bet he didn't go along!'

'Yes, he did actually.' Will remonstrated.

Becky looked at him sceptically. 'You didn't have to get drunk though did you?' She sneered.

'Here we go again.' He said sadly as he made his way toward the door. He paused before leaving the room and waved at Becky who had resumed drying her hair. She switched the dryer off once more and looked up at him with irritation.

'I'm not hung over if that's what you think!' He said.
Becky responded by flicking the switch again so Will tried howling over the noise.

'I'm dying because I spent all night fighting off those fucking dreams again!'

'I thought you said you'd gotten over all that!' She bellowed back.

She was right because he had said that. But what he'd meant was, he had gotten over taking them seriously, he was still dreaming them night after night. They were nonetheless intrusions and they came with just the same ferocity with Thom appearing just as tangible to him now as he'd ever done.

Thom could still spook him but he no longer saw him as the caricature monster of nightmares as he had before, but rather as a simple foible of his overzealous and over informed imagination. He might still jump up sweating in the night but it was such a relief knowing them for what they were. He would often sit up for a while and curse quietly until he was calm but now at least he could lie back down and wait for the new day.

Ideally, he would stop dreaming the fucking things altogether. It left him so deprived of sleep but sometimes while he lay awake in the darkness waiting to nod back off it left him the space to think about some of the other objects he'd taken from his dear old mum's house when they'd cleared it out.

It was a lovely surprise finding Matt's old books like that. He'd been amazed at first that his mother had kept them, she had never been one for either sentiment or clutter, but he knew now she wasn't as indifferent to that part of the past as she had liked to convey. In fact, Will liked to think his mum had treasured the books just as much as he did now.

But it was the stuff in the gramophone case that really made him think long into the night that became dawn.

It intrigued him enormously. Would had saddened him immensely too if he didn't make an effort to drown the sorrow with waves of curious fascination.

There were a lot of official papers in the box, her last Will and testament, Matt's birth certificate and his death certificate.

She was so brilliantly organised with bills and stuff that that sort of thing was never really going to shock him. The other things he'd found however, certainly did.

The stuff about his dad had really thrown him, left him breathless for a while. He had to sit back down on his mum's bed when he first saw the yellowing piece of print and was so pleased that Becks was occupied in another room with Penny so she hadn't seen the colour drain out of him.

He wasn't sure how he felt at the time other than numb with the shock of it. So when he had finished sifting through everything else inside he simply shut the case tight and made sure he told Becks that he'd locked it.

It had made coming across his mum and dad's wedding photos difficult.

They were still in pristine condition, hidden away in soft white envelopes and then he found the wedding certificate and a plastic horseshoe wrapped in its own fading ribbon.

When had she decided to lock all of those things away?

Why had she decided to move from their home and their friends and go to live in Highbury? Never to see anyone they knew ever again?

Though the memories were vague, he still remembered the Christmas parties he and Matt had attended. Once dressed smart and uncomfortably and another time in just their jim-jams, crawling excitedly between legs, ladies on the couch smoking cigarettes and laughing noisily.

So his parents had had enough family and friends.

He remembered an Uncle Jack with greased-back hair who would pretend to steal the boys' noses by pinching them between his fingers and showing them his thumb. If he had been a real uncle there had been cousins too. Boys a bit older than Matt who liked to wrestle you and a girl who might have been the wresters' sister, always threatening to tell on them.

From memory they had never seen these people often but why didn't his mum and he ever see any of them ever again?

110

Was she ashamed? Did she just run from their fuss and their help? She was always one to shun attention however well-meaning and if they really were family or even half decent friends they would have tried to help surely?

So, Will would wrack his brain trying to remember other facts and other names and if he was really lucky it was enough distraction to have tricked him back to sleep.

James didn't know what to think to be honest. He couldn't even begin to tell you how he was feeling emotionally. Probably have to describe himself as dumbstruck for the moment, as good a word as any really. Would need to give the news time to sink in before he could begin to rationalise and deal with the disappointment.

Completely flabbergasted had been his immediate reaction when the young lady had explained. He hadn't had any riposte whatsoever, just sat there for however long studying her face for inspiration. He could clearly see it had made her uncomfortable but there really wasn't anything he could do for the while, he'd been so dazed.

The poor thing, wasn't her fault at all. Just the messenger but he'd pushed her and pushed her for an acceptable reason and she'd finally caved in and told him. Just to shut him up he imagined and how thoroughly successful she'd been.

It was difficult to fathom, how a thing like that could get in your file in the first place let alone remain there for so many years maligning career and reputation.

James had tried to explain the whole thing to Brian as best he could. If nothing else he hoped it would help him come to terms with it by spouting it all aloud, might even make it less ludicrous.

He had taken a decent enough bottle of the blended stuff with him to compensate his friend for being the sounding board of his latest upset. Brian had a bit of a chest as well and had clearly welcomed the medicinal benefits of the whisky and once his friend had found a couple of dubious looking glasses and they'd sat down James began his explanation.

It was just a matter of weeks after Debbie had finally persuaded him to hang up his chalk blotter when there had been an accusation by the mother of one of the better equipped boys that James had helped a number of his pupils' cheat with the written part of their projects which contributed a significant amount of marks to the exam totals.

The mother clearly objected to the thought of her son being deprived of the glory of exceeding all others, if only academically.

'You see some of those kids were marvellous on the practical side of things. Could strip an engine down with their eyes closed, greased monkey's some of them, but they weren't so hot on the written word. To be honest a few of them struggled to write their own name.'

'So, you gave them a wee bit a help.' Brian reasoned.
'I did,' James declared, 'although I wouldn't except that anyone cheated as such... there was just a little bit of plagiarism.' He admitted.

James had fished out some old papers from a previous year and had distributed photocopies to those who required them. The idea was for each of the boys to formulate their own S.A. using the information.

'I'd been doing it for years,' he said defiantly, 'simply to give the less academic lads a chance.'

'Of course, the Head had to perform an official investigation as the Education Board would have had to have been informed of the complaint. He was quite sympathetic, unofficially speaking, but he did the investigation thoroughly, interviewing the accuser and some of the accused, myself included.'

James waited for Brian to light a cigarette and fight off the coughing fit it provoked.

'None of the accused said anything particularly damaging,' he continued, 'but at some point, the S.A.'s the boys had submitted were gathered together and gone through and of course a couple of the lazy sods had just copied the script from my photocopy.'

Brian looked at James gravely through a cloud of smoke and shook his head.
'Anyway, shall we have another dram?' James suggested, 'I could really do with calming down.'

Both men drank noiselessly but for the wheezing of Brian's chest. Then after a few minutes contemplation and another top up to his glass James reflected on how little the episode had entered his thoughts at the time.

'You see,' he told Brian, 'by the time the investigation was in full swing I had already secured my new position outside of teaching and was already looking towards a whole new chapter.'

'Well no one can blame yer for wanting out.' Brian said. 'Could'nee be easy with your first wife there and all.'

'Oh no, you see,' James explained, 'I'd already left the school where Veronica was working… well I had to, or felt I had to and Debbie was at home by now carrying our first child. I'd only been at this particular school for about eighteen months so I hadn't really built up much of a relationship with anyone. No one to fight my corner once I'd gone you see.'

'Sentenced in your absence then.' Brian said. 'So it would seem.'

Brian shifted in his chair and lit another cigarette. 'What will'ye be doin now then?' He asked.

'Do you no, I haven't the foggiest! I hadn't really made any plans other than to teach again.'

James paused abruptly and Brian noticed how pale he had become as it dawned on him that his prospects were virtually nought.

Brian must have sensed his thoughts or perhaps he saw the film of moisture across his friend's eyes because he grabbed the bottle of whiskey and waved it in front of James to snap him away from his stark musings.
'Come on man,' he said, 'to hell with all that and let's have another drink!'

****

The woman's voice went straight through him. He didn't dare move his head. If he moved it he just knew it might implode. But there was that nauseating aftertaste of whisky billowing from the back of his throat and if he didn't prop himself up he'd be sick or it felt like he would.

Oh, and those fucking people in the corridor having some sort of argument at god knows what unearthly hour in whatever primitive dialect they were using.

Why couldn't they just fuck off quietly to their cleaning jobs or their hot dog stalls and allow others to get some sleep?

Slam went the door, even louder than usual: Someone's final word on the argument he hoped.

Relative silence for a moment then slam went the door again. James clenched his head at the temples to quell the pain the vibration had given him.

It was at times like these he wondered why the bloody hell he carried on. If it wasn't for the sake of the children he really would wonder.

Now he needed a trip to the loo, but at this time of the morning there was bound to be a queue and he hated hanging around all unwashed and of course there would be all the different smells to endure.

He pondered the knowledge of how Brian solved the problem; but really there were limits. Brian even had the gall to proudly explain how he always rinsed the bottle out afterwards, as though he were being stringent in his hygiene bless him.

That was how you became, James supposed, living on your own in these circumstances for any length of time.

Anyway, didn't want to dwell on that scenario, especially with the teaching opportunity gone. He could quite feasibly still be here himself for quite a while and to be honest it hadn't taken him very long to get into the habit of sniffing his clothes for freshness before putting them on.

Nevertheless, he hadn't reached the stage where he felt comfortable with the idea of pissing into a bottle and couldn't put it off forever. Somehow, he had to crawl out of bed and put some clothes on so as to go and have a pee.

Probably need to do something to himself on his return too. A hangover always seemed to release the primitive urges toward self-abuse.

You couldn't for one moment believe Brian didn't do the same or didn't also try to squeeze the result out into that bottle of his.

****

By mid-morning James had given himself a shower and dressed himself having finally shaken off his black mood.

He felt awful now for berating the poor Eastern European's like that in the morning, who were merely trying to make something of their lives through honest hard work.

If James sometimes felt he was given the thin end of the wedge he'd just have to try and imagine how awful their previous existence had been, what with the war and all of the side effects war brought with it.

So, in a nutshell he resolved, it was time to stop feeling sorry for himself.

He was taking himself off to the labour exchange and then he'd buy the local paper to look at the jobs being advertised.

Miraculously, Debbie had only taken her usual sum from the account for the second month running; so, James was going to have a look in BHS to see if he could get smartened up a bit for whatever new career lay in wait.

You see, he reassured his reflection before he set off... there were plenty of reasons to be positive if you bothered to look for them.

Becky sat at her vanity unit having dried her hair. According to the clock Will was already twenty minutes later than she'd hoped he'd be. Although he wasn't actually later than he'd said he'd be it was just she couldn't help but worry. He was still tied up at work the last time she phoned, but how many times in the past had he used that as an excuse?

She'd made him promise. He said he could handle it and he'd bloody well promised.

Jules already had enough to cope with just introducing them to her new fella and so Becky watched herself getting more and more agitated in the mirror.

She bloody meant it this time! He had better not be too late and he had better not have been drinking!

She'd seen it so many times lately, Will, embarrassing everyone by rolling up late, pissed and stupid.

If he's too late we won't even bother going, she decided, as she pawed her way round the mound of cotton wool in front of her in search of the lighter that had rolled somewhere in that direction.

Having found it the tiniest ripple of guilt passed over her, having officially banned smoking from either of the bedrooms but then it was lit.

She turned and breathed a plume of smoke in the direction of her dress hanging there on the outside of the fitted wardrobes and hoped it wasn't going to be too much for that bloody awful pub where they were meeting Jules. Becky hated being conspicuous.

It had annoyed her a bit that Jules had wanted to have a drink beforehand even though it was she who'd chosen the Mandarin Palace for the meal and knew the restaurant didn't have a bar to rendezvous in.

It didn't give them much choice but to meet in the Kings Head or that big pub in the middle of the roundabout that seemed to have its name changed almost weekly in the hope of discarding the old name's reputation. It was the sort of place where it was easier to get a fight than a drink and if Jules wanted this fella to get a good first impression of where she'd grown up they had to stay well away from there.

Now having looked at the clock again Becky had changed her mind and was actually relieved that the scenario of creeping sheepishly up to a dining table where Jules and her new beau might have been patiently waiting for too long was gone. It was much less awkward just walking into a pub late.

'Although if he's not home soon we really shan't be going.' She muttered anxiously to herself as she rolled the cigarette carefully around her crystal ashtray.

For the want of a distraction she once again scrutinised the clump of eyelashes in the mirror where she thought she may have applied too much mascara then stretched her eyelid in a bid to separate the worst hairs.

Becky wasn't one for wearing a lot of make-up usually, which was probably for the best, considering the lack of skill she had in applying it.

Now did she have time to take the mascara off and reapply it? As she pondered the thought ash from the cigarette had formed and fallen onto the quilt long before the need to catch it had dawned. Furious now, she dispensed with the problem of her appearance and began to do what she could to discard the mess she'd made.

Where in god's earth was Will anyway? He still wasn't officially late yet, but couldn't he, just for once in his life surprise her and be early?

He'd mentioned Clive had wanted a quick word with him before he left the office and now she wondered if he'd just made that up so he could have a couple of crafty drinks? Or perhaps he'd say he had to have a quick drink because Clive had left him exasperated or he'd have to have a drink because Clive had decided he was doing well again or perhaps he'd even have to have a drink because Clive had invited him and he couldn't turn him down.

Well she'd heard all of those excuses before and she'd made him promise not to use any of them or any of the other countless shitty little stories tonight, so where the fuck was he?

Becky picked up the elegant designer watch with the tiny plain face that Will had presented her with on the previous Christmas.

A quarter to eight at the latest he had told her and now it was seven thirty-six.

She was beginning to feel a chill sitting there in just her knickers and bra and contemplated putting on the dress if she could summon up the courage to trust him and anyway it wouldn't hurt to stand around ready as the chance of him having a shower and changing was long gone and they would have to go immediately when he eventually appeared.

Well, actually she changed her mind and he would have to wait the two minutes it would take for her to slip on the dress.

For the moment she would just have another cigarette instead. This time in the living room as there was too much of a risk of being caught now.

The phone rang from every aspect of the apartment. Becky's heart sank. She felt a slurred excuse waiting for her from some indistinct venue somewhere in the City.

'Hiya.' Came a familiar voice.

'Oh, it's you.' Becky said, unable to conceal both the relief and disappointment.

'Why? Who were you expecting?' Julie's piercing tone questioned.

'Will.'

'Oh god isn't he home yet? You won't be late, will you?'

'No, I'm sure we won't,' Becky lied, 'it's probably just the trains.'

'Oh god, *please* don't be late!' Julie implored, 'that King's Head is a right dive!'

Becky thought quickly.

'If we're not there by half past Jules we'll meet you in the Mandarin.'

'So, you are going to be late!'

'No!... look... I don't know, I'm just saying if the worse comes to the worst we'll have to meet you in the restaurant so you don't have to hang around for us.'

119

Julie could hear the strain in Becky's voice and moved to calm her down.

'Oh well... I'm sure Mark won't mind.' She said.

'Yes, well, you don't know how long they'll hold the table for do ya Jules... what time did you say you booked it for?'

'Half eight.'

'Well there you are then... we'd better meet you in there.'

'Okay then hun.'

'Okay?'

'Yeah... but please don't be too late.'

'We won't darling.'

'Okay, speak later!'

'Yeah, see you then.'

Becky replaced the receiver and got up from the bed. She suddenly shivered, feeling the goose bumps spread across her shoulders.

She was going into the other room to have a ciggy and wrap herself around one of the big cushions.

She shifted herself to the end of the bed and stretched out her profound legs in the direction of the door but now her vision was blurred. There was something in her eye that couldn't be ignored. It would need cleaning up and re-applying after all, then the thought of that, her ridiculous fucking makeup again, ruining itself because of him. She'd tried but Becky couldn't fight the tide of her disappointment.

'Grow up!' She moaned at her indistinct reflection as she sat back heavily on the bed.

The tears began to flow, tears and eyeliner that she could taste on her lips, but it wasn't happening because she wouldn't let it happen and she felt herself sneer at the thought. This wasn't her and she wasn't going to let it be her. Not just the slightest thing, the slightest crisis, she was a married woman now for Christ's sakes' and you dealt with these upsets didn't you?

She was cold and she had got herself all flustered worrying about Jules and this new guy who Jules really liked. Wanted it to work out for her this time, was desperate for her, but that didn't give her the right to get angry and upset and take her frustrations out on Will did it?

Did she really have to keep reminding herself about what he was going through? Was she really that thick or that thoughtless?

Will was still so mortified by his mother's death that he couldn't even acknowledge it and he was beginning to slip over the edge. If she'd actually bothered to think about it properly, as in really think about it, she would have been a proper help to him. Then in that moment she'd had some kind of epiphany.

Becky suddenly decided it was about time for her and Will to have words. She sniffed the moisture away and gasped.

She was going to sit Will down and tell him what she wanted. The pussyfooting around him was going to have to go. It hadn't done him any good, to let go of the strings. He'd only started to unravel.

From now on she wasn't going to let him get blotto every night like he had been and she wasn't going to let him stay up all hours reading all of those history books like he had been. No wonder he was still having those bloody dreams when he was adding fuel to them.

She was going to explain to him he was going to have to start being a lot more reasonable if he didn't want her to turn into a battle-axe. Show her a little bit of respect and stop being selfish. It was bound to get a reaction of one sort or another. Either way he might actually stop for a moment and take stock of his life and if Clive or the job or whatever it was at work was getting too much for him he would have to look around for something else. She'd made up her mind.

Having stubbed out the cigarette Becky made her way back into the bedroom still pondering her new tough stance.

See the trouble with Will she thought, was that he was always pushing himself so hard. What with reading the history stuff and spending hours doing research for his job he might not get to bed until past two o'clock. It didn't leave him too many hours left to sleep.

121

It was a wonder how he found time to have nightmares to be honest.

Becky's mum reckoned Will was burning his candle at both ends just so he didn't have to deal with his mum's going and the nightmares were proof to her that the stress of it all was getting to him enough to even make her fret about his health.

Becky had agreed at the time. She had agreed but that was all. Now she was actually going to do something about it.

Jules being Jules put all of Will's problems down to him drinking too much. Becky knew there was some truth in that too and more than anything else she was going to nag him and nag him into cutting down.

Becky lifted her dress down by its hanger and gently smoothed the delicate material with the palm of her hand.

That was another thing, she decided. It was all very well her telling Will to stop obsessing about his job but she hadn't stopped spending the money he was making had she?

The dress and the shoes together had cost the best part of three hundred pounds and she'd barely batted an eyelid.

There you are then... another thing she was going to do. Economise.

It was actually quite a pleasant thought. Something practical they could both do that was bound to ease the pressure.

If Will objected to the idea she'd tell him straight, that it was him she loved and not his money. She meant it too, she really did. She'd be happy to live in a tent if she had to just as long as they were together.

Of course, she had to concede, it was easy enough to say that when you knew things were never going to be that bad but it was conceivable enough that they may not be able to afford the lifestyle they were leading now. It was no big deal as far as Becky was concerned. They could do without half of the things they had and they would still be doing very well. For a start, they didn't need two cars and Will certainly didn't need the Aston Martin he'd ordered. They hardly had the chance to drive anywhere anyway.

Not with-standing that, they could buy a three-bedroomed semi in some parts of Hornchurch with the equity they'd made on the apartment and they wouldn't have any of the extortionate management fees that went with it. Fuck paying for that swimming pool anymore.

Will would probably sneer at the suggestion. He just spent money willy-nilly and much more than that he wanted people to see him do it. He was always showing off really; a bit more subtle then some but all a bit offensive anyway.

She would often remind him that her parents had always lived comfortably in a three- bedroomed place and she hadn't had anything to complain about when she was growing up. It was ridiculous to think otherwise. She'd been really happy.

Of course, there weren't many kids who had to live the sort of childhood Will had, but that was nothing to do with money or going without things, he'd said so himself. In fact, she could never understand how much he strived for the material things when it had never even seemed like he enjoyed them once he had them.

Becky pulled the dress over her shoulders and wiped away the stains from under her eyes.

It looked nice she thought, but she would definitely have to take the mascara off and start again.

The clock showed it had gone a quarter to eight but somehow, she'd stopped stressing too much now. She would have to see out this evening and hope to god Jules would be fine with whatever happened.

****

Will noticed a movement. Someone in the building opposite was putting on a jacket and was about to leave his office. He scanned the whole floor and found this bloke to be the last one in there then he looked around his own floor and found the main desk empty. Clive had already gone and all that were left were a couple of the IT guys doing the evening backup.

It was Friday evening after all and that's what people did on Friday in this weather. They either raced home to their Surbitons for a bottle of wine in the garden or they gathered outside the pubs and wine bars of the City and enjoyed the last rays of sun that reflected golden on every pane of glass and ripple of traffic.

Will's team had gone down to the Embankment for a drink on one of the pub barges. The Thames and the view of Parliament, a very pleasant notion in his mind, but he and Becks had this awful dinner party to go to with Julie and her new guy, god help them all.

He'd insisted he wasn't going to go at first, but Becks had worn him down. He couldn't understand why she still bothered. She knew he couldn't stand Julie and it was more than obvious that the feeling was mutual.

'Do it for me.' Becks had asked and he'd grudgingly agreed. Had to really with the way he'd been behaving recently, but now the evening had come he'd wished he'd been a little more obstinate. Becks would have been sceptical if he'd told her he'd been held up at work, but unfortunately for him it was true and he'd been locked in Clive's office while the scrawny bastard pawed over his spec book like the proverbial headmaster to Will's naughty schoolboy.

That was the way of the future apparently; Every Friday afternoon for the foreseeable future according to Clive.

Will knew he should feel humiliated but somehow, he didn't. He just felt exhausted. Numbed by the calamities that were beginning to close in and suffocate him.

All he wanted to do now, to do ever, for that matter, was to drink himself to oblivion before his job, his debts, Clive and those fucking ridiculous visions he was having took him there.

Will shook his head and loosened his tie.
He looked back over at the building opposite. His office friend had gone.

Glancing at his Rolex he knew he had better make a move himself as Becks had dared him to be late and for a change it would be nice to avoid that scenario before meeting up with people with the pair of them shrouded by an unspoken atmosphere.

The Reuters screen was blurred now as he scanned it and he fluttered his eyelids rapidly until the columns became focused then he flicked his desk key to lock away his daybook and slipped the key into a side pocket of his jacket which had been crumpled on the back of his chair since lunchtime.

On his way down in the lift he looked deep into the mirror. He was pale and tired. There were wrinkles forming around the dark bags below his eyes and he thought about Thom again. Now there was a face that needed help. But where had that face come from? Will urged his reflection to come up with the name of an acquaintance or a character from television to match the old man. Images formed in Will's mind then quickly dissolved as he dismissed them as unsuitable.

Jeffrey Bernard, a friend's father, Scrooge. Close in some ways but not right.
Thom wore the same sort of nightdress as Scrooge though, but of course Scrooge didn't have all of those disgusting gashes on his neck.

Will's mind switched off the guessing once he'd found himself at the revolving doors in the lobby.

Queen Victoria Street was empty. The coaches were gone and the traffic had diminished to a trickle of saloons and black cabs. He sauntered across the dusty road in search of a cab with a yellow for hire light and didn't have to wait long on such a warm evening.

The cab swung back under Blackfriars' Railway Bridge then turned toward the length of the deserted Queen Victoria Street. Will spied the giant dome of Saint Paul's through the gaps in the buildings as it turned to the colour of rust under the blaze of the setting sun.

The traffic increased significantly as the cab headed down through King William Street and on toward the Bank.

Will glanced at his watch fretfully. He'd really hoped there would be time for a quick short before he got on the train. He wouldn't even have ordered ice. But even if there wasn't the time on this side of the journey he was going to make sure he had a bloody good drink at the other end of the line. After all the shit and anxiety he'd put up with over the last week, the least he deserved, he decided, was a bloody good drink. In fact, there was half a chance he might get pissed out of his head tonight.

Becks could hardly blame him considering he was going to have to put up with Julie all night, especially on top of the week he'd had.

They'd probably all get pissed anyway unless Julie's new bloke was one of those who didn't mind driving or worse still actually wanted to drive. Petrol Heads wasn't it? Boring idiots.

Will wouldn't even be able to mention his Aston if this guy was like that. He'd take it over. Will didn't know anything about cars.

The whole bloody evening suddenly sounded unbearable. That was it then... a quick change of plan. He would have one or two very swift drinks before the train and then he'd have an even quicker livener when he got indoors before Becks had the chance to smell his breath.

The taxi finally drew up at the end of Old Broad Street behind the station.

Will handed over a note then made a point of pocketing all of the change as he still had a gripe with all black cab drivers.

He lit a cigarette while he contemplated where to have his drink. Somewhere close obviously but somewhere you could actually get served with a bit of haste.

The Railway Tavern opposite the taxi rank was besieged with suits all across the pavement so wasn't even worth thinking about. He looked along Liverpool Street to the White Hart on the far corner. It seemed a lot less crowded outside which, he decided, was good enough.

He walked in the middle of the empty road, toward the Great Eastern and looked through the grimy windows of the hotel bar which wasn't busy, but he still remembered that awful night he and Becks had spent there which was why it hadn't even hit the radar of his thoughts to go there and now his eyes were fixed on those revolving doors as he approached from the opposite direction he and Becks had arrived from that night.

Will wondered if he would see anyone going in or out as it wouldn't be busy on a Friday evening with the business guys going home for the weekend and it no longer being the place to shag a stranger.

Still reputations did take a time to be lost as Becks first comments had proven although it must have had a more discernible clientele in the past because just beside the entrance doors Will noticed a rectangular blue plaque, the sort you found on a lot of the older buildings in the centre of London, usually depicting the name of a famous former resident. So the place must have been respectable to begin with. Will had never noticed it before. It was a lot lower down the wall than most of them seemed to be. He tried to read the narrative with a languid interest as he passed. Couldn't really make it out from where he was so he snaked between two parked cars to take a closer look.

He read the words on the plaque quickly but it was enough for the information to register like a sharp blow to the head.

Will winced and his eyes flickered with incredulity as he read the words over again and again.

SITE OF THE FIRST BETHLEHEM HOSPITAL 1247 - 1676

They were the same words each time and however hard he may have wished for it he hadn't made a mistake.

He'd read about the place in the books he'd bought. The hospital had been mentioned in all manner of publications, even Pepys, that famous diarist from the seventeenth century had visited there. The place they incarcerated the mentally ill or just the downright deranged, all living in squalor, chained or left to their own devices.

The byname they'd used then was still well known in Will's lifetime.

Bethlehem Hospital was much better known as Bedlam.

Will could have screamed and perhaps he did but he was far too bewildered to be sure and now his arms and legs began to convulse and seized him with panic. Panic that coursed through his arms and struck at his heart which was leaping uncontrollably to the point where it seemed it might fail. It truly felt as though he was about to die and he tried desperately to call for help but he could barely breathe and now his heart lurched and his balance was gone. Will grasped at the pavement as he buckled and fell upon it.

Chapter 20 – The morning after the dinner before

The telephone rang again. Becky's heart leapt with anticipation but it was only Jules.

'Hiya.' Becky said in a clearly disheartened tone.

'Still not home then.' Her friend surmised.

'No.' Becky murmured almost inaudibly.

'Has he phoned yet?'

No, he hadn't.

'Oh Becky.' Julie sighed.

Becky didn't reply, she couldn't she was choked up now.

'He's such a little fucker!' Julie pronounced fiercely.

She could hear Becky fighting back the tears and sniffing up her snot.

'I'm so sorry.' She said.

'Don't be,' Becky finally managed to say, 'and don't worry about me, I'm fine.'

'You should try and get some sleep Becky.' Julie advised. 'Have you told your mum yet?'

'No.' Becky replied shaking her head determinedly.

'Are you gonna?'

'Not yet.'

'Well if you need me to come over babe you just have to say you know?'

'I know… thanks mate. Has Mark gone home then?'

'Yeah he has… I'm gonna get some sleep meself now.' Julie snorted lewdly as she remembered the previous night's exertions.

The two women had had a very different time since Julie's new boyfriend had dropped Becky home after the restaurant.

The first thing Becky did as they drove through the gate and into the car park was look up at the apartment in the hope a light would be on but it wasn't. She knew Will wouldn't have gone to bed so he still hadn't arrived home or worse, he'd got home, found it empty and had gone out again.

She couldn't help regretting going out herself now.

Heaven knew how hard she'd resisted the invitation but it was such a kind gesture of Jules and Mark especially, to keep on at her until she'd agreed to join them. She just couldn't turn them down as they'd been so insistent and as Jules had said and they'd all thought at the time Will was going to turn up later anyway wasn't he?

Mark had made everyone feel so comfortable considering how awkward it could have been for all three of them gathered around the table.

Becky had expected to spend the whole evening making discreet glances at her wrist watch willing her idiot, selfish husband to appear but it wasn't like that at all and there were even parts of the meal when she'd forgotten about his absence or at least hadn't cared.

It had been nice and she was so pleased for Jules because she could tell how much she liked Mark.

Obviously there came a time when it was better that Will didn't show. Jules must have thought that as well because she knew what Will could be like as the evening wore on. Might really have embarrassed everyone if he was properly drunk.

Now on reflection Becky could have handled that. She could have handled him being paralytic and falling all over the place just as long as she knew where he was.

Had he been calling home while she was at the restaurant?

It was nearly eleven o'clock in the morning now and still nothing from him.

She didn't know what to do and she was just... so very tired.

What time had it been when she'd started calling the hospitals? Three, was it?

She'd called the emergency services first and had got a right royal telling off for using their number. It was directory enquiries after that and trying to remember the names of hospitals across London. Saint Thomas's, Bart's, Whitechapel, Whipps Cross... she'd called them all. All the ones she could think of anyway and then she'd checked the local ones and it didn't seem he'd been admitted anywhere thank god.

There were police stations as well to consider knowing what a prat Will could be, but wouldn't the police have made him call home?

Becky had just sat there all this time biting her nails and smoking cigarettes while she still had some.

The first time Jules had called she thought it had to be Will as it was so early in the morning, but Jules had just wanted to check that Will had got home and more than anything, Becky guessed, to tell her that Mark had spent the night. Not really a surprise knowing what Jules was like but Becky would still like to hear all the details some time once Will had come home safe.

Will crouched back on his haunches and needed a hand pressed hard against the pavement to steady himself but it wasn't going to last and now there were passers-by.

He needed shelter, he could feel the impending doom pressing him down as if the sky was about to collapse and with it the full force of Thom's prophesy bearing down upon him... upon everyone everywhere.

He leapt back up in one wild movement and the need to become hidden and out of daylight's reach propelled him toward the pub where he had first been heading.

He needed a drink; lots of strong drinks.

It almost felt like he was going to collapse his heart was pounding so violently. It was hard to catch his breath and could the others on the street see him shaking? He was just, well... he was fucking *trembling* with fear, but he kept walking, hunched to make himself less visible from above, less of a target.

He got himself past the small gathering under the hoardings outside then he was in amongst the crowd of the saloon bar, submerged among shoulders all clambering for the attention of the bar staff.

It was so fucking hot but he had to stay with it and if he was shoving he was sorry, he didn't want to invite trouble, he just needed a drink 'cause he was fucking terrified!

By the time he was finally served his shirt was clinging to him. He opted for four large whiskies, no ice and he downed one immediately at the bar. He would have downed them all if there weren't so many punters waiting to cut in. He struggled out from them all with the glasses clenched between his fingers and palms and put the glasses down on a high table already fully laden with drinks.

'Sorry.' He said to the girls perched on the nearby stools, but he wasn't really sorry because he wasn't going outside again, not until the booze had a chance to work its way through his bloodstream.

He was going to down his drinks and smoke a cigarette right there at the table as there wasn't a space anywhere else.

The second whisky was swallowed whole and he lit his cigarette. It didn't sit well in his stomach but he caught the resurgence in his mouth. There was nothing else to do but pull hard on his cigarette and steel himself for the next drink. It stayed down better this time and he could feel the alcohol having some effect thank god.

One of the girls threw him a dirty look. Fuck her Will thought as he stubbed out his cigarette in her ashtray.

He swilled the last whisky around its glass but couldn't make it any bigger. What would he do when it was gone? He didn't want to fight his way back to the bar and now the girls were being joined by a guy, shimmying his way through the bodies with two glasses of wine and a spilt pint of lager.

Okay, he thought, swallow the last drink and walk toward the door. Didn't have to go out... he could look outside and see how it made him feel first. At least it would be cooler.

There you are then Will thought as he stood under a canopy and lit another cigarette. The alcohol was working.

He needed to contemplate what he was going to do now. Still didn't feel confident that he could make it home without freaking out again... and what then?

What was he going to say to Becks? How was he going to behave with her? How was he going to try to behave?

He couldn't burden her with his discovery.

He stood awkwardly among more strangers. What was he going to do? What? Will was at a total loss... he couldn't think... he just... and it had happened, he had suddenly choked up, exhaling a slight wail that he caught in the palm of his hand and there were a few tears shed that had bled through his fingers.

People around him had noticed it so he felt he had no other choice than to move on.

He remembered there was an off licence in Houndsditch. So, he went there.

He bought a bottle of Glenfiddich at a premium, but what did money matter now?

He certainly got some strange looks from the Asian guys behind the counter when he went back into the pokey little shop to buy some more cigarettes. The screw top was off the bottle and they may even have witnessed him taking a swig just outside in the street.

He was outside the shop again now on the narrow pavement holding the bottle in one hand and a cigarette in the other. He was getting strange looks from everyone now, pedestrians, motorists, all of them.

Couldn't stay on the street like this in the city, it was too out of place. He needed to go to the West end where every fucker walking around at night was some sort of oddball.

Will hailed a black cab. It seemed like he'd never stopped using them since he'd sworn to never get in one of the things again, still once more, what did it matter in the big scheme of things now?

The driver wasn't happy when he noticed Will clutching the whisky but Will promised he wouldn't be touching it while he was on his journey. Not that there was any chance of getting a tip in the first place but now the cunt was going to have to scramble around on the floor to pick up his fare where Will was going to drop it.

'The Strand.' He'd said when asked where he wanted to go. That would be alright. If he got dropped at the far end by Charing Cross he could decide whether to make his way left toward Soho or right toward Covent Garden. Either way no one was going to notice him swigging from a bottle there. It was going to be busy though on such a warm evening. The thought itself left him deflated.

Now though, just as the cab had passed Australia House at the end of Fleet Street, he thought of the perfect place to go.

He had the driver take him to Trafalgar Square and set him down by the arch at the mouth of the Mall.

He dropped a ten pound note thoughtlessly into the driver's hand and made his way into the Mall's relative calm.

The headlights didn't follow him as he made his way behind the tall plane trees and down the sloped lawn between the flower beds and toward the lake in the darkness of St James's Park.

Lights glinted on the water but there was nothing there to guide him, just dense black pockets all around, on the lake and to either side as he walked. He may have thought such obscurity would spook him but somehow, he found it comforting. It seemed a good place to hide.

As he warily made his way down he felt the earth become hard underfoot and decided to just sit down there on the dewy grass.

He pressed the palms of his hands against the turf and rubbed the moisture between his fingers.

Will knew he'd better start slugging on the whisky to drown the detail of what he was doing.

He took a couple of quick swigs and felt the burn rise inside him then he lit a cigarette and hid the glow of it in the cup of his hand. The last thing he needed was to get caught by the Park Keeper or by the Old Bill. He didn't want to be moved on. He really needed the time and the space to think.

Another deep slug of the single malt made him feel better if only a little sick.

After a short time, Will looked around him as his eyes adjusted to the conditions and he could make out a little of the detail surrounding him. The void to his right had now become a dense thicket of branches and leaves. There wasn't any colour on view from what he could see so there wasn't anyone sleeping rough in there it felt safe to surmise. That was a relief, he would have had to move then... show whoever in that situation some respect.

Another few slugs of the whisky and another cigarette, head swimming a bit but it had made him a little bit more at ease.

So what was he going to do now? So, what the fuck was he really going to do?

He couldn't just sit there with a wet arse getting pissed without actually thinking of a plan for the future, otherwise what? Fall asleep and wake up cold and hung over with the same fucking problems? No one could help him with them... he'd be like Thom if he said anything... they'd lock him away.

Becks would even lock him away because she would think it would be helping him.

Will clenched his eyes and his fists and fought back the surge of despair that had suddenly engulfed him.

That fucking Thom had ruined his life! Why the fuck did he pick on him? He spends the night in a shithole of a hotel and gets his head... *sneaked* into by some fucking mad parasite and now any normal life was gone... over!

Then what about Becks? What the fuck was this going to do to Becks?

He couldn't stop all of the tears coming and now there was snot all over his face so he loosened his shirt from his trousers and wiped himself dry with its tail.

He wanted to scream or to run somewhere but he couldn't. It was too fucking bad... he was going to have to stop all the tears and think of something.

Will took the comfort of the whisky and lit another cigarette. Just needed to calm down and stop freaking out and drink some more fucking whisky.

'It's alright.' He mumbled to himself after he'd drunk again. 'You're gonna be alright... stay calm.' And it seemed to be working. 'Just stay calm.'

Will stared out toward the twinkling reflections on the lake. He was almost tempted to lie down but he knew that would be a mistake. He had to do some thinking first.

What was it that Will could do in all practicality?

He had to think closely about the things Thom had been telling him all of this time to try and find a thread of hope. Something he could get involved in to try and prevent the catastrophe that was going to befall them all.

But in reality, he knew it was useless. If he were a politician then maybe he could try and pass a motion opposing whatever it was the morons in Whitehall were going to carry forward that would spark the end, or if he were in the forces? Being in the right place at the right time? Not to follow the order to push the button or to be there to shoot the officer who was going to give that order.

This was stuff of delusions. What the fuck could some Mickey Mouse softs trader do to change anything but the short-term price of cocoa? Chocolate bars might jump by ten pence but that wouldn't even get Alan ready for war. Anything he tried to do would just be futile.

Will groped to the side of him for the box of cigarettes and was going to light the next one with the one he was still smoking.

It just didn't make sense that Thom had reached out to him with all of the people who must have come and gone in and out of that hotel room over the years. Was it just fate?

Will put the new cigarette to his lips but before he moved to light it he felt a sudden sense of elation moving upward through him making his body tingle.

That was it! Suddenly he'd comprehended that Thom had actually *targeted* him. It wasn't fate at all! Thom had plagued him because he knew Will could actually get himself in a position to influence things. God knew how but if this man could send visions of himself forward hundreds of years in time to seek him out why would it be such a big ask for him to find the right man

Will had sort of picked up on it earlier when he'd been trawling his memory on the things Thom had ranted about but he'd obviously discarded it up until just when the thought about how useless it was to be a softs trader had given him the thought.

Still true, course it was, but to be an *energy trader* on the other hand and to have an influence on the crude market could make a massive difference; an enormous difference... and who knew? Maybe even *the* difference.

Thom had mentioned oil a number of times. Course, he hadn't used the actual word but he had said something about fighting for the Moors treasure. Well the Arabs didn't have any treasure other than oil did they? The food that fed the new beasts as Thom had called them. Oil was what fed the beasts and the beasts were the machines weren't they? The cars, the boats, the planes...

If there was ever going to be another large scale, global sized war it was going to be about oil. That was why the Iraqis had taken the gamble on invading Kuwait and that was why the Kuwaitis had taken the gamble first by slide drilling into the Iraqi oilfields.

It was just the start of more and more conflicts as the crude became scarcer and the price rocketed higher and higher until it became unobtainable by any means other than force.

Will finally lit the cigarette then shakily held the whisky bottle before him.

'I'm gonna do it.' He mumbled out loud and jerked the bottle skyward before taking another draft.

Time passed slowly for a while just sitting there in awe of his epiphany. Then with a sudden call of nature Will clambered up and made his way gingerly to the nearest bush to piss. No one had jumped out thankfully, no homeless, no couple in lust, no badgers; he made his way back to the same spot and sat back down then hung his head in quiet contemplation.

He wondered how difficult it would be to get a transfer onto the Energy desk?

Didn't know the head honcho too well but he was sure Clive would go for it. He'd probably jump at the chance to get him off of the softs desk.

It would only be a sideways move on the surface. Will would have to find a legitimate reason for wanting to make such a move. Everyone in the City wanted ambition. It would take him some further thought but it was doable.

How much did he know about energy anyway? First thing Al would ask, but Will knew some to be fair. He knew the exchanges they were traded on and he knew the contracts, the Brent and the WTI crudes and the gasoils. The cash trading was a complicated business but if he were just to be doing the hedging he knew he could do it. A futures trade was a futures trade at the end of the day.

He'd have to knuckle down once he was in though, learn the markets thoroughly, gain the trust of those he would be working for, knock the drinking on the head... speaking of which... Will lifted the bottle and shook it gently, he felt something at least sloshing around inside. It wasn't much but he raised the bottom skyward and savoured all that was left.

Now it was empty.

****

Will wasn't sure how much longer he'd stayed in the peaceful darkness of St James's Park. Might have dozed for a while but he didn't think so. It would have suited him very well to have stayed in that same spot for ever but he still had a home to go to and the most perfect wife who he loved with every single ounce of himself, every minute part of him and he was going to have to suffer the agony of witnessing her disappointment again for spoiling a dinner party, for leaving her on her own, for leaving her frightened for his safety... for breaking a promise.

He could have easily have loitered a little longer than he should have on the red thoroughfare of the Mall as he marked the beauty of the palace in the distance while the glow of the headlights approached and widened at speed but he had a duty to stay alive and to get home and to try in some way to make Becks feel better... for a while at least.

Just so drunk and so tired and he'd probably been crying again as his eyes stung so much when he wiped them. How ragged he must have looked.

He did at least ditch the bottle in a basket by the lake before he walked back through the arch into Trafalgar Square with his damp trousers creased around his knees and his collar up to fend off the chill in the breeze.

He hoped to find a night bus around the square. He had taken them in the past from outside the National Portrait Gallery.

There were crowds of people mulling around, a gang of skinheads looking for mischief too. Will needed to avoid them fuckers.

So what bus was it he had to catch? He didn't want to be trying to read the little information panels that they had on the bus stops themselves, not with those fuckers standing right by them. Probably couldn't focus on the tiny print anyway. He decided he'd wait to see where one was going and if it was in the right direction he'd get on it.

There were still the normal buses running but there had been one go past with the letter 'N' preceding its number. That meant night bus, 'N' for 'night bus.'

Still all in all there were too many buses Will decided. It was far too confusing and there were too many skinheads as well. He thought he'd move on and try and find a phone box that hadn't been jammed by the druggies so he could call Becks.

He staggered around the corner and up along the Charing Cross Road wobbling a little as he walked.

The first bank of phone boxes he came across had the usual stench of urine. Two didn't take coins and the third took the money but didn't produce a dialling tone.

He found his cigarettes and lit one. Just a couple left so he decided he'd better find a convenience store further up the road or off toward China Town.

The place he found seemed to stock everything on its dirty shelves, strange vegetables that looked ripe toward rotten, packets labelled in Chinese, all manner of liquor bottles and exotic beers, scotch too but just the blended. Will bought his usual box of cigarettes and resisted the warm booze.

He was thirsty now more than anything and he needed a proper drink to quell the sourness in his mouth. Something ice-cold, didn't even have to be alcoholic but if it was, wonderful. The hangover was already knocking on the door.

He was in Lisle Street and smoked his way between the lost tourists and the dumper bins of the restaurants, jumping between the street and kerb to avoid vehicle and pedestrian in turn.

Now he found himself on Wardour Street. This was more like it! Right toward Oxford Street and left down to Leicester Square.

He took a left where he knew he could get a coke and a burger even if he couldn't get a beer and if that turned out to be the case he would take away the food and drink in a bag and he would go home to face the music.

Sod trying for the night bus again, he'd go down to Charing Cross Station and get one of them unlicensed cabs that were always touting for business, recognizable by the black faces of their drivers and the dented front wings of the cars.

Another cigarette and another bunch of obstacles to bypass then he was in Leicester Square with its swarms of nightlife and lowlife.

Didn't know where to start first, he could get moved on by the bouncers outside the Empire nightclub or he could see if he could find a seat on the benches inside the square and scout his surroundings in comfort. But the gates of the square were closed. Will gazed around in search of somewhere else to go.

There wasn't much that he could see, so that was it as far as he was concerned, he'd take a walk around the other side of the square to the Burger King, get an enormous coke and maybe his own body weight in burgers.

As he walked purple lights behind smoked glass caught his attention, some sort of a wine bar, but he could see it was winding down. He looked back toward the square and now he saw a girl standing by the railings holding a guitar.

For some reason he headed straight toward her with some pace in his stride, he didn't know why but perhaps it was just that she looked interesting, simply that and perhaps she might be fun too.

Once he'd reached her Will stopped abruptly, legs splayed, a wide grin on his face.
The busker quickly stopped playing by caressing the strings tightly with the palm of her hand, showing her slender fingers, dirty and bitten around their tips.

The memory of the tune she had been strumming was gone from him in that instant.

She was smiling at him, not so much with her mouth but with her dark eyes.
He was going to ask why she was wearing a woollen hat on such a night as this but as he focused distractedly on the clumps of brown hair on either of her temples he found himself asking if she did requests.

'I've already got somewhere to stay if that's what you mean.' She said softly.
Will grinned again.

'No, I just want you to sing me a song darling.' He explained. 'It's the end of the world as we know it... R.E.M.?'

'That's just a lot of shouting apart from the chorus.' She sniggered.

Will laughed because it was true.

'Then can you play something else that might cheer me up?' He asked with a wry smile.

'Oh, I *thought* you were sad.' She said. 'I could tell even though you were trying to look happy.'

'Clever.' He said.

'Why is it the end of the world?' She asked with concern.

'It just is... I mean it really is unless I can do something to stop it from happening.'

The girl looked at him wide eyed.

'I found out something awful today,' he said solemnly, 'and now I'm supposed to save the world and that ain't good.'

'Are you a spy?' She asked in earnest.

'No darling,' Will chuckled, 'I'm not a spy. I'm not an anything really, but I've got to start trying to be soon.'

'Do you want me to help you?'

'How's that?'

'Help you do whatever it is you need to do.' She said.

'Oh.' Will said with a sigh. 'Thank you sweetheart but I'm not doing anything tonight 'cept getting a burger and going home.'

He took the cigarettes out of his jacket and struggled to get the lighter to work.

'Do you want one of these?' He mumbled with the cigarette between his lips and waved the box in the girls' direction.

'Not now.' She said, taking Will a little aback with the suggestion the two of them were going to be together for some time.

Having finally lit his smoke he threw out a great plume to mark the achievement.

'Can I buy you something to eat then?' He asked valiantly.

'If you want to.' She said.

'I don't suppose you eat burgers do you?'

'Yes.'

'Oh you do? That's a surprise; I thought you'd be a vegetarian, you kind of look like one if you don't mind me saying?'

'No, I love meat.' She replied as she bent down and picked up the handful of change that had been thrown into the guitar case before carefully placing the instrument inside and zipping it up.

The unlikely pair weaved their way together toward the welcoming lights of the restaurant on the other side of the square.

There looked like a horribly long queue inside as far as Will could tell but once the girl had barged her way through with her guitar he could see it wasn't that bad after all.

He ordered what she'd asked for and told the server to make it two of the same. He was ravenous now to be honest but he didn't want the girl to think he was a gluttonous pig so he'd make do with the paltry cheeseburger and fries. It was the cola that he truly needed anyway.

'I was supposed to go out to dinner with my wife tonight.' Will confessed as they waited for the food to arrive.

'Won't she be worried?' The girl asked, unfazed by the revelation.

'Yeah, she'll be worried and she'll be sad and she'll be angry.'

'Poor her.' The girl said as Will took hold of their bags of food and they turned away from the counter.

'Where do you want to sit?' He asked.

'Not in here,' she said, 'I want to tell you about what me and my friends have been doing to save the world too... sort of anyway, at least to stop it getting even more polluted.'

She lead Will out of the square and along a passage with traditional restaurants that were having their al fresco furniture packed away by grubby waiters wearing their respective waist coat uniforms, then moved right along a narrow street which took them behind the portrait gallery.

Will had virtually finished his drink by the time the girl came to a halt.

'Here.' She said, motioning Will with her eyes toward a set of steps covered by a low archway before balancing her guitar between the top step and a wall. Then she sat carefully beside it.

142

'Why here?' Will asked unimpressed.

'It's just private and it's clean.'

'Fair enough.' Will concluded as he handed over her meal.

'Thank you!' She said as she opened the bag eagerly, 'I come here if it's pouring down or if I can't get home.'

'Right.' Will replied unwrapping his own burger.

They munched their food quietly, Will scrutinizing her soft features as she chomped away absentmindedly.

'Where is home?' Will asked when he had finished eating.

'Islington.' She said.

'With your parents?'

She held her hand across her mouth to suppress her laughter and stop the mouthful of food she was eating from falling out, shaking her head rigorously to express the negative.

'Don't laugh!' He cooed. 'I didn't think someone who busks for a living was going to have her own place!'

'I don't.' She said narrowing her eyes in readiness for the expected derogatory remark.

'Flat share?'

'Sort of,' she agreed 'I live in a squat with fourteen other people.'

'Right.' Will said with a slight air of amusement. 'And your boyfriend yeah?'

'Not anymore.' She answered sadly.

'No?'

'He was murdered by some drug dealers.'

'Oh fuck, I'm so sorry!' Will gasped in dismay.

'Yeah.' She said nodding her confirmation.

'Fuck!'

'Yeah.' She said still nodding.

'I don't know what to say darling, that's just...' Will searched his surroundings with his arms stretched out wide trying to pluck words worth saying somehow from the air around him.

'You know... look that's... fuck!' Was all he could muster. 'That's awful... and how long ago was this?'

'Christmas.' She murmured.

'Fuck!'

'I kept telling him to stop taking drugs.' She stated casually as she finished her fries.

Will fumbled for his cigarettes.

'Go on have one.' He offered, reaching out the box to her as if in some way it might comfort her.

'Thanks.' She said leaping to her feet to take one.

Will struggled once more to make the lighter work. Gallantry was finally abandoned as he handed his new friend the instrument hoping she may be more successful.

Their fingers brushed in the hand over and Will was taken by how small and delicate hers were.

She was shaking the lighter now in her dirty grip and for those few moments he was stood close beside her bearing down over the woollen hat that covered her sharp little head and with her eventual success they both gathered around the flame, his hands cupped around hers.

'Wish I could buy you a drink...' He said softly as she looked up at him. 'But there isn't anywhere open.'

'I know a place.' She said.

'Not a disco?'

'No.' She answered and she was smiling again.

'Well let's go then.'

'You don't need to I'm alright,' she assured him 'I'm getting used to it.'

'But I want one.' He said.

'And it's really loud... probably louder than a disco.'

'That's fine,' he said flicking the butt of his cigarette onto the pavement 'as long as they'll take me and I can get a drink.'

She could tell by his stance he was ready to move immediately.

'Okay,' she said, 'only I thought you wanted to talk about the world and everything?'

She picked up her guitar ready to move.

'What do you mean?'

'You know,' she said with a sigh, 'I thought you might want to tell me what you're doing... you know... to change things and that.'

Will looked at her perplexed.

'You know, changing the world, saving the planet, if you were serious!'

'Oh, trust me darling I'm serious.' Will answered as they began walking back toward Leicester Square.

'Good,' she said, 'because I really wanted to tell you what I was doing too you know?'

'So, tell me.' He said reluctantly.

He knew his tone had given him away but she seemed happy enough to take up the invitation to talk.

'Some of the guys I live with have been squatting for years,' she enthused 'and they always find these big mansions that have just been left empty for ages and reclaim them for people who need somewhere to stay.'

'People like you.' Will observed.

'Do you still need to go home?' She asked.

'I do yes, but I don't want to.'

'Well if you need somewhere to sleep you can stay there with me.' She suggested nonchalantly.

'Anyone is invited as long as they're not addicts, or you know... proper winos.'

Will was holding the bag with all the waste and unfinished drink cartons. He was busy looking for a bin to put it in but there didn't seem to be any around and now he was back listening to her as they walked.

'My friend Gill,' she was saying, 'who I met when we were trying to stop the M11 link road getting built; she wants me to go up with her to Manchester to stop the second runway. She was at Greenham for over a year...'

Will was trying to keep up with the conversation but had been distracted by someone shadowing them at a distance; A young man in a scruffy brown jumper with curly hair to match. He smiled and nodded when Will stared straight at him.

'Alright chief!' He thought he'd heard him call but Will had decided to ignore him.

Will followed his busker friend past the spot where they'd met and out of the square and back onto Wardour Street with the Chinese restaurants empty.

There were still a couple of Toms half-heartedly touting for business from a narrow doorway. Will just managed to tug the girl toward him to prevent her from treading on something regurgitated that was snaking its way down on a stream of disinfectant from the back of the restaurant on the corner of that section of Street. She was still talking continuously, oblivious to anything around her.

Will was becoming irritated now and he really needed to get to a drink.

The boy in the jumper suddenly appeared from between a couple of rickshaws.

'You alright chief?' He asked again cheerfully.

'What do you want?' Will groaned with disdain.

'Just wanna see where you're going.' The boy answered.

'Right, fuck off!' Will warned him and pointed out the length of the road. Unperturbed the boy grinned mischievously. Will immediately clouted him over the head with the bag of waste and let it fall onto the street as he kept moving.

The couple continued walking leaving the boy behind clutching his head but still with that inane grin.

'He's an idiot.' The girl said in disgust.

'You know him then do you?' Will asked with some indignation but she didn't answer.

At the junction with Shaftesbury Avenue they waited to cross. 'There's too many cars.' She said.

It must have been that last remark that pushed Will's level of frustration over the line. He suddenly felt he couldn't let it go.

'I know so many things you don't.' He barked. 'I really have to find a way to do something and not just spend my time talking about it!'

She turned abruptly just as she was about to cross, her guitar swinging wildly from the handle.

'What do you mean?' She asked.

146

'You know,' he said, 'people like you wearing weird hats and talking about peace and love and all that, having your riots in Trafalgar Square because you don't wanna pay the fucking Poll Tax!'

She was staring at him in bewilderment now.

'You don't do anything, you just sing songs and moan about the traffic!' He spat.

He pulled out his cigarettes and tried to light one with the lighter which now might really have run out of gas. He shook it violently a number of times and eventually it sparked into flame.

'The trouble with you people,' he mumbled through the gap left by the cigarette in his mouth, 'is you're all so fucking naïve.'

He looked up then to see her reaction but she'd moved. He spun around and looked back down toward the square but she had gone.

'That's it then!' He shrieked up toward the sky. 'You run away as soon as you don't like it! ...it's me who'll do it all... by myself!'

Then he lowered his voice to almost a whisper, the next words sounding ridiculous as he thought them, even in his condition.

'I'll save the world.' He said.

He stood there a while afterwards with the pedestrians keeping a discreet distance as they passed.

'Help me someone,' he murmured, 'please help me Becks.'

Will turned the key to his front door, his hands steady for once and the operation was more or less silent.

Becks would be in bed.

They always slept in late on Saturday morning and Becks, bless her, would probably have stayed up half the night waiting for him to come home or at least call her.

God! she had to be in bed! He just couldn't face her disappointment now.

He crouched down and slipped off his shoes then the blood swam around his brain making him all the more light-headed and nauseous.

The plan was to have a large gulp of something strong then sneak into the spare room to take a quick look at one of the books that had some maps in there showing the streets of London back in Thom's day. He just wanted to see if Bedlam was on them anywhere. Nothing more than that because any reading he did for the foreseeable future was going to have to be about the oil markets.

He'd have a sleep then if he could. Just slip his clothes off and get under the quilt and hopefully he'd be in a better frame of mind to deal with Becks in a couple of hours' time. He was going to have to stay in control and not fall apart on her.

Will had been so concentrated on the careful movement of his feet it had taken a time to realize he was being watched and when he raised his head he was shocked to see Becks standing there quite still beside the far sofa.

She stood upright watching him sternly, something intensely serious and distant in her expression.

Why also was she dressed so early? Properly dressed with her hair immaculate?

On reflection Will calculated it must have taken him a good ten seconds before he saw the suitcase.

Becky finally spoke, trying to sound stern but her voice cracked as the stream of words she had been rehearsing from the moment she had put down the phone to Jules and thought of her desperate plan began to spill out across the room. Words in curious waves and tone as if she were still only imagining the scene that had somehow been forced upon her. The thing she was doing right now, the risk she was about to take for herself but most of all for Will to hopefully shock him into his senses were the things she had to explain. Then she was picking up the small suitcase and walking past him toward the door.

Will had listened, his head bowed with shame and he hadn't said anything, had barely raised an arm to stop her and then when he did finally speak he said the most hurtful thing she thought he could have said.

The bastard asked her if he could help her with the case. At least it gave her the final spurt of determination she needed to bat away the hand he had extended as it reached out toward her own hand on the handle of the case and drag the thing down the stairs by herself. It even felt quite easy to lift into the boot of her car. She was so fucking angry! So fucking humiliated, so very disappointed, but she wasn't going to let him see her fall apart.

She walked steadily to the drivers' door and slipped inside. He wasn't going to see how broken he'd made her but she couldn't resist that one last peak herself. She adjusted the mirror fully expecting him to have followed her down to the car park or at least, at the very least, be looking down at her from the window of their bedroom. But he wasn't there.

Becky started the engine and drove out through the gates, away from everything that had mattered, but she didn't get far, she had to pull over. Couldn't drive through the tears, she just had to let them come and keep coming and then when it finally felt like she could manage she turned the engine on again and made the short journey home to her mum and dad.

Will was still standing where she'd left him in a state of suspended animation. If he could just stay there as he was without ever moving again it felt like he could handle it.

Who could blame her? He couldn't quite believe he'd had the strength to let her go and wasn't even prepared to entertain the thought that he was too weak to fight for her to stay. He was saving her from so much more misery. A fucking hero he was.

She was everything of course. She was still everything, but it would be so much easier to face what he had to do alone.

So for now and probably forever Becks was gone.
The rush of grief was flowing right through him and he could feel the familiar ache he used to get when he was a child return.

He had really hoped sometime not that long ago that he wouldn't ever have to feel that dull pain again but sure enough it was there.

For now though, just for now, he was going to stay standing exactly where he was.

James sat cross-legged on the bed. He had taken off the only decent pair of slacks he had left and hung them in the wardrobe. Other than that, he was still in his vest, shirt and socks.

If he felt the urge he could simply slip the slacks back on and he'd be as good as ready to go out.

He was still so restless you see. It had been a good couple of hours since he'd taken the boys back home but he was still angry with himself for saying some of the things he'd said to Adam. Scott had listened too but anything you said to Scott that didn't involve wrestling or whatever other mindless rubbish Deborah was happy to let the boys watch seemed to go in one ear and out of the other with Scott. He was of course that much younger too.

Adam on the other hand seemed quite perplexed. He went very quiet very quickly and seemed to have an almost disapproving expression on his face from that moment on.

James could see his mother in him quite distinctly sometimes. He really shouldn't have let himself get all riled up just because the boy was showing loyalty to his mother who after all was being attacked, fairly in James's view, if only with inappropriate timing. But really Adam should be commended if anything for being a loyal son. Something James felt sure would be reversed should his mother have any harsh words about him, although James was fully aware that Deborah wouldn't be so crass as to recite a list of her grievances aimed at him in front of the children. She could play a terribly good game that bitch.

Still the whole reason for James making such an ill-judged outburst was because she was being just too difficult lately. The woman couldn't be any less accommodating if she had tried whenever James tried to have anything at all his own way.

There were those tickets for Brands Hatch for instance. Okay, it was only rally car racing but child tickets were free and adult tickets pretty damn cheap compared to what they charged for the Grand Prix, but she'd blocked it of course, wouldn't swap her Sunday with his. He'd told her he couldn't have given more notice because he hadn't known about it himself until the Tuesday when he'd called her, but she wouldn't budge and she wouldn't even give him a reason as to why not. She didn't have to explain herself to him was all she'd said, which was fine, but James couldn't help point out that the boys were losing out because of her bloody mindedness.

Seemed to stick where it hurt that one, which was probably why she'd done what she had with this bloody film that he couldn't take them to see. She knew only too well there weren't a huge amount of films suitable for their age that he could take them to see on a fortnightly basis which was why he had to seize every opportunity when it became available. It was one of the very few activities affordable to him for heaven's sake. Bowling or ice-skating cost an absolute fortune.

Yes, he could take them to the park if the weather was half decent but just try to get them to enjoy themselves for more than ten minutes when there was a howling wind blowing you numb with cold.

Of course, he would have loved to have taken them to the library but he only ever got to see them of a Sunday.

He was still bloody furious even now. That film was his to take them to!
It had only started showing the week before but the bitch had gone and gazumped him by taking them then.

Then you would have thought the boys would have mentioned it? Well of course they didn't, not until the three of them were already in Romford and heading toward the cinema complex.

Adam, bless him, tried to be helpful, said there had been a whole lot of children's films in last week's trailers and he didn't mind which one he saw as they had all looked good. But then James had to explain that when they say 'coming soon' in these trailers they could mean next month or even several months later rather than the following week and unfortunately James was proved correct. Out of the ten or so films posted up on the board there was only the one the boys had already seen the week before and one other that they would be permitted to watch given its unclassified rating

152

but judging by the content it was still essentially an adult film that they wouldn't want to see.

So, there they were the three of them, sitting glumly in McDonald's while James racked his brain for something else to do without coming up with a single idea. He just hadn't enough money with him for the pricier alternatives.

Then somehow, he had looked at the beautiful unblemished faces of his boys, which seemed so despondent that they didn't even appear to be enjoying their burger meals and he just sort of lost control a bit and began to rant.

'This is all your mother's fault!' He heard himself remonstrate much too loudly.

It didn't stop there either, oh no, it just carried on and on. The Brands Hatch day they were forced to miss was mentioned, how the bitch wouldn't lend him his own fucking car for Christ's sake! So, he could take them places and right through every act of meanness and he really meant right through.

He even brought up Peterborough where 'Listen boys, you could have stayed the whole weekend with daddy'... and onwards through all of the other terrible, rotten things their bitch mother had done to him.

That was what was making James feel so bloody restless now as he sat half naked on his bed. His stomach was quite queasy with remorse and self-disgust.

He would never have imagined he'd be one of those parents who'd drag his own children into the dark melee left when things became so acrimonious between man and wife. That he could scar those poor boys by feeding them even a glimpse of his own sorrow was unforgivable.

He couldn't bear it. Just couldn't bear thinking about it anymore. The anxiety it was causing him was actually making him shake. He would have to get out. Take his mind off things.

It would, he thought, be helpful to displace a little of the angst he felt with a friend and perhaps hear a few words of reason. A little joviality wouldn't go amiss either if it were at all possible.

It was easy enough to slip the slacks back on and then the shoes and just slip across the hallway. The foil being the offer of a quick tin or two, and Brian, bless him, as at most times proved to be his usual compliant self.

'I just need to nip down to the Spar and I'll be back in a jiffy.' James explained with a new found zeal.

Brian watched James disappear from site and closed the door. He stood motionless for a minute with eyes closed then with a heavy sigh went about preparing the room for his guest.

Becky hadn't been out after work since she'd moved back in with her mum but then Jules had said it was hardly going out if you were just going round a mates' house for a curry and a chat.

So, there she was sitting on Jules sofa clutching a glass of Pinot Grigio while her friend tried to hunt down the takeaway menu she thought she kept buried away somewhere in her odds and sods draw in the kitchen.

Jules had been really supportive since the breakup even if she did put her foot in it sometimes, but she knew Jules, it was never out of meanness saying some of the things she said, it was just that she was thick.

Anyhow it was so nice of her to go on and on at her to make her come round. She must have known she wasn't going to be much company. She was still, you know... sad.

As soon as she turned up on the doorstep and Jules had let her in the tears had started.

Jules had shrieked when she saw her because of the amount of weight she'd lost and it wasn't one of those nice sounds your friends make when you'd been trying to lose weight or you looked nice, it was just shock really. Becky knew how dreadful she looked. She was just so tired and washed out and then when Jules had grabbed her and hugged her like she did Becky couldn't stop herself from being in floods there and then on her shoulder even before the front door had been closed.

Jules hadn't stopped making a real fuss of her since then, getting the wine for them both and making her promise she was actually going to eat something once they'd ordered it.

Becky wasn't at all hungry really but she'd promised anyway. She knew Jules was trying to look after her. Made up for some of the thoughtless things she said like the other evening on the phone when she'd been gushing on about this new guy Mark and she'd actually said how strange it was that she'd finally connected with someone just as Becky had broken up. Becky knew she didn't mean it like that but when she put the receiver down and went up alone to her old bedroom for the night she was just really, really down.

Didn't matter now and she just hoped Jules and Mark would make a real go of it. Jules never seemed to hold onto them for long and it couldn't just be because she was always jumping into bed with them straight away because Mark was still around.

Even so, that was Jules main problem Becky had realized, everything seemed to revolve around sex.

Becky still hadn't forgotten that other time Jules had called her when she brought up the idea that Will might have spent that night he had gone missing with someone. Jules just didn't think and what could she say to her? That it hadn't crossed her mind? Or just that she hoped he hadn't? Anyway, if she had seen the state of him when he came home that morning she wouldn't have thought anyone would have gone anywhere near him. He looked like he'd spent the night in the cells or on a park bench rather than in a bed.

Becky still trusted him anyway.

'But what would she do if he had?' Jules had asked.

Couldn't answer that... she still loved him so maybe that was the answer?

That question was just so typical of Jules's mindset. She seemed to view men like they were the enemy a lot of the time and she always seemed to be trying to catch them out or was trying to score points off of them instead of getting to know them properly, relaxing, having fun.

But then perhaps she was the last one worthy of an opinion Becky thought as she looked deep into the swirl of wine in her glass without wishing to drink it; breaking up within months of actually getting married for gods' sake.

It was just such a bloody waste.

Everyone had been so surprised but what choice had he given her?

There'd be someone else the girls at work had told her just to try and make her feel better. But there wouldn't be... she already knew that.

They had been soul mates... Becky and Will... Will and Becky.

She and Will had been completely relaxed in each other's company and they definitely had had plenty of fun together.

She suddenly thought back to that time the other summer in the apartment when there was a heat wave and they couldn't sleep and they were dying it was so hot. Will didn't even have an alcoholic drink which was saying something.

Both of them had spent the night drinking pints of iced water trying to get cool but that didn't seem to help much then Will jumped up out of the blue and suggested driving down to the coast even though they were already in bed.

'What naked?' She'd joked, but then Will had persuaded her to put on some underwear and sneak down to the car with him. He was only wearing his boxers and a pair or trainers so he could use the pedals and she was just in her bra and knickers.
They drove all the way to Southend like that waving at anyone who looked in on them.

Will nearly crashed the car a couple of times because she kept grabbing at his gear stick every time he changed up or down on the real gear stick and they were both just *killing* themselves laughing.

It was the sort of happiness Becky had always dreamed of and doing things like that with Will made her feel like she was in a film sometimes.

Poor old Jules had never found herself in that situation so Becky wouldn't even contemplate confessing those sorts of feelings to her.

Now she felt she really needed a cigarette and she was going to have one even though Jules didn't like it. She'd given her a saucer to use as an ashtray so she may as well take the opportunity while she could.

God only knew what Jules was still doing in the kitchen? She couldn't even hear her swearing anymore. Might even finish it before Jules appeared again and might even start on the wine now. Give Jules what she wanted and everyone knew it was easier to talk when you'd had a drink.

At least she knew Jules would be supportive about what she'd done. Mum hadn't been... well she had but she hadn't. She was fine at first about her going home but she thought it was just a tiff that had got out of hand and would be over in a couple of days. Becky had too to be honest. Thought Will would come crawling after her but not a word.

Even dad was worried and he'd actually said that they should both at least talk about it, but wasn't the onus on Will to get in touch? Wasn't she the one who'd been wronged?

When Jules eventually appeared with the menu she found her friend hunched over herself with her shoulders shaking up and down and a hand across her face quietly sobbing.

Brian sighed, a heavy sigh before turning down the volume knob of the radio.

'Hold yer horses!' He shouted as he trudged over to the door.

'It's only me!' James gasped as the door was opened.

Of course it was thought Brian, who else would it be?

James stood before him gaunt faced with red-rimmed eyes.

'Come on then.' Brian said sharply, turning back towards his chair.

James entered and clanked the door shut heavily behind him.

'I'm sorry to intrude,' James gushed, 'but that woman is an absolute fucking bitch!'

'She still giving you the what for?' Brian asked wearily.

'She still won't let me see them!' James complained. 'Not until you start providing for them she said.'

James made his way over to the bed swaying slightly as he went and placed the supermarket bag he'd been carrying carefully onto the grimy quilt and plonked himself awkwardly beside it.

'I see yer ahead o'me again.' Brian remarked coldly.

'It's that fucking woman!' James groaned. 'You've completely wiped the account of every penny I had I told her... and now I'm to somehow miraculously produce more!'

Brian rolled his eyes to show his disbelief.

'Then get yourself a job she said!' James continued. 'But that's all I bloody well do I told her... look for a job that doesn't exist... You know how hard I've tried don't you Brian?'

'Aye.' Brian replied dismally.

'Why don't you try McDonald's? She said, McDonald's are always advertising for staff... Could you see it though Brian? A fifty-three year old man with a Bsc standing behind the counter of a burger bar?'

'Jus' pour yerself a drink.' Brian said as he shook his head with affinity.

'Oh, I've brought my own tonight.' James replied triumphantly as he wrestled a large plastic bottle from his carrier bag.

'Cider.' He announced holding the bottle up to show Brian the label.

'My god, but you're dredging the barrel now though.' Was Brian's response.

'One pound sixty-nine for two litres.' James offered as a defence.

'Aye, but It'll rot yer brain that stuff.' Brian remarked plaintively.

'Beggars can't be choosers.' James countered as he inspected the inside of a mug.

Well at least it'll save my brew for a change Brian mused.

'I mean what does she expect me to do? James resumed, 'I'll just keep on trying is all I can do. But in the meantime, the children will still need a father. She isn't even thinking of the children... I've kept a few pounds you see Brian, to take them out to the pictures or something... or bowling. They wouldn't need to go without fun if she were to let me see them... I'm the only one going without, you know yourself, don't you? I've been having breakfast cereal for breakfast *and* supper for the past week to allow me to take them somewhere.'

'She's a mean'un alright.' Brian concluded.

'Do you know she wouldn't even let me speak to them over the phone?' James gasped having just swallowed a sizeable draft from the mug.

'She said they were playing. Well of course they were playing: it's what they do on Saturday's. All bloody day in fact, so I'm sure they wouldn't have minded breaking away from whatever they were playing for a few minutes to speak to their father... they must wonder what's happened to me.'

'Then ye know the path yer have to go down don'tcha!' Brian said abruptly because he'd said the same thing on countless occasions now.

James had to get the courts involved now, that was Brian's way of thinking. He needed to start thinking about legal access. He could understand James's apprehension about dragging his kiddies through the courts, of course he could; but at the end of the day what other choice did he have?

The man had to start acting like a man instead of forever whining to him and drinking every drop of whisky he might have in the place.

Chapter 26 –The Crack up

The first weekend when Becks had gone was nothing more than a blur now.

He slept that first night without even Thom for company and he'd slept for hours and hours, right through to Sunday afternoon. The remainder of the day was spent quietly on a couch with the vague comfort of cigarettes and alcohol.

He contemplated how brave he would need to be but had to spend much of the time berating himself for the tears he kept crying.

Didn't eat because he couldn't eat, but the worst thing was when he went to bed that night he couldn't sleep except for a very short time when he nodded off from sheer exhaustion. Even then that fucker Thom had him awake and blindly searching for his wife on the empty side of his bed.

He still got up for work on the Monday morning, dizzy with tiredness, but full of resolve to begin his plan.

He was going to speak to Clive the very first chance that he got to find out what could be done about a move to the Energy desk.

The idea was to play it cool as best he could and explain that it might be beneficial to everyone if he could have a fresh start. Happy to take a step back and do some execution work until he was back in the groove. Use all of the bullshit phrases Clive lapped up to make it seem plausible.

He was even content to concede that it was fair for him to have taken all the losses on his own account. In all honesty he was willing to say and do pretty much anything that would get him the move.

There was still one dry cleaned suit hanging in his work wardrobe and three ironed shirts to choose from, all thanks to Becks and her smart housekeeping.

He could take his own clothes to the dry cleaners and he could probably remember how to use the washing machine, but he wouldn't have a clue how to contact the ironing people, Becks took care of those sort of things. Anyway, that was another hurdle that would have to wait for the time being given how there were far more important things to occupy his mind.

When he'd dressed he gave himself a full inspection in the mirror and although he was looking decidedly pale and pasty the rest of the image stood up well enough. He could have given the brogues a quick shine but all in all he was satisfied.

Having checked all of the appliances were off and the windows were shut, as they both used to do, Will left the apartment.

He should have double locked the door as per usual but he hoped if Becks came back on the off chance she might just see it as a sign that he wasn't turning her away from what was rightfully hers.

He made his way through the ornate gates of the apartment block to begin the short journey down to the little station halt to catch the shuttle train that would take him onto the full rail network.

He was fine when he'd left but suddenly he had a hollow feeling in his stomach that was much more than hunger yet his legs had gone the opposite way. They were heavy and awkward to move as if he wasn't fully in control of them.

'Fucksake.' He mumbled as he plodded along self-consciously with the sun on his face.

His fellow commuters ambled over the iron bridge facing him as they did every morning, but rather than slip seamlessly between them as he normally would have and make his way down the ramp to the platform, Will hung back and fiddled in his jacket for his cigarettes.

He just wasn't comfortable with the way he was walking and he didn't feel able to do the customary exchanges he and these familiar strangers liked to engage in, even if it were just a nod of the head or a simple 'good morning.'

He'd smoke a cigarette and keep his distance.
When the train came he quickly made his way down the ramp to catch it using the handrail to steady his unreliable footsteps before boarding the carriage at the furthest end where he could be alone.

It was an awful start to the day.

Stop being a prick and pull yourself together, was all he could think of as he attempted to give himself a firm talking to.

A short time later when the train had reached its destination Will resolved to let all of those before him go, completely forgetting those waiting for the opposing journey were waiting to board his carriage.

He fought his way against the tide of people who by their expressions were obviously unhappy at having to wait for him to exit; and to think he was going to try to save those fuckers lives.

The hand rail which ran all the way up the steps and over to the London platform was a lifesaver now as his legs grew heavier with every footstep.

He couldn't think what was wrong other than needing to confront Clive and he'd been alright doing that before, admittedly not over something as crucial as this, but at least he knew exactly what he was going to say.

Standing at his usual spot on the platform he lit another cigarette and the sensation was almost like he could feel the smoke swirling inside him feeling as empty as he did.

It suddenly dawned on him that he was actually frightened, he couldn't really understand why and that seemed to make it all the worse. He was even having trouble catching his breath now so he tossed the cigarette down onto the tracks.

He thought for a moment of turning back and going home to the apartment but he couldn't, how could he? He needed to see Clive, he needed to make progress... he had to get on the train.

Will saw the lights glimmer in the distance, then the train came into view as it edged the bend in the track.

His heart was already pumping and his throat began to tighten. Empty train he tried to reassure himself. Own seat so don't worry, but his heart began to beat much faster and the tingling that came with it began to stretch from his chest to his arms.

'Don't.' He muttered almost audibly while all the other passengers were already shuffling nearer to the edge of the platform where the doors would open.

Shouldn't have smoked... idiot... struggling to breathe.

The train slid to a halt and the crowd readjusted its position to align with the doors.

Deep breathes Billy boy. Hands tingling now but look, everything's okay, lots of seats... own seat by the window so no one's going to look at you.

He was almost the last to step onto the carriage and he was fine once inside. It was really quite cool in there so fine, but then came the bleeping noise of the doors as they shut behind him.

Now he had palpitations; he jerked his hand toward a rail and grasped tightly because it felt as if his heart was practically doing flips.

He was shaking now, hands visibly shaking and he really couldn't breathe.

Calm down, he pleaded with himself. Take deep breathes... everyone looking over now.

Palpitations and surging pains in his chest and all along his left arm, he held the handrail tighter but now his legs were beginning to falter. He spread them apart and held on for dear life. Oh fuck! Because now he was forced to screw his eyes shut to fend off the tears.

Didn't think he could bear it any longer. Heart bursting, couldn't catch breath... going to die on a *fucking train!*

But then just as he was certain the final moment had come the panic seemed to dissipate just a little bit and he managed to catch his breath.

Calm down arse! He reprimanded himself. Not going to die, just get a fucking grip! Deep breath... that's it... hold it... and... see no one looking now, evading eye contact or asleep.

Sit down now he urged himself, only a twenty-minute journey wasn't it? No, not even that now with the train just passing Becontree. Only about fifteen minutes or so; go sit by the window he repeated in his head.

Deep breath... that's it... good boy, soon be at Barking.
See you can do this, he admonished once he'd settled into his seat. He was still shaking but he was slowly getting back in control. There was no-one watching, no-one making him uncomfortable. He could

relax now, or at least try to relax. He just had to sit still and fix his eyes on the back of the seat in front of him and block out everything else. Better still, he could just close them. Yes, it was better. He was managing.

The train was approaching Barking station now. If he was lucky he might not have anyone coming to sit next to him. He could sit in the first seat to make it awkward for anyone to join him, but then why create a fuss if someone was just sitting beside him? He couldn't be dealing with any sort of fuss now.

Soon the train had slowed as it edged along the platform. Fucking hell look at the crowds! Was his immediate reaction and in that same moment the palpitations started again and with a vengeance, he could feel his windpipe beginning to close. Will ran a sweaty hand over his face.

The train finally ground to a halt. More people at his end of the carriage than usual but not as many as he'd expected when he'd first seen the crowd. He was alright he decided as the doors opened... yeah... but what would he be like when the doors closed again? It would be like last time only worse!

Perhaps he should get off? He considered as he watched the new passengers find seats, yet no one seemed to be coming over as far as him so might just be alright.

Sit up straight he resolved. That was it. Probably no more than twelve minutes left on the journey anyway. He could stay on for that.

The doors closed. Slow steady breathes he coached himself. Will looked out of the window as the train moved off. There was a thin strip of sky above the concrete overpass to his right and for some reason he was relieved to see some cloud cover.

Nothing to worry about now he decided even if he was still shaking like a leaf.

He promised to buy himself a cup of coffee once he reached Fenchurch Street; something to look forward to, grand size, proper Italian.

His breathing was much easier now, in and out of his nostrils, slow and even.

He was going to be fine, one way or another he was going to get to work and who knew? With all the effort he was making perhaps he really would get the job in Energy.

The train passed the Canary Wharf building in the distance as it moved ever nearer to its destination. That big chunk of concrete and steel, Will thought, all to be swept away if he didn't do something about it. There's your focus he resolved and it seemed to be working.

He was soon at Fenchurch Street buying coffee and then he was on the tube in the heat and among serious crowds.

It was too hot down there and everyone was crushed against each other trying to manoeuvre where they could find space.

When he had edged past everyone at his stop a gust of gritty air swept through Will's damp locks and he could feel the moisture beneath his shirt bite cold against his skin.

He didn't know how he had survived that part of the journey through the searing heat and suffocating intensity of the cramped underground network. Maybe, he thought, he was so busy dealing with the physical challenge of keeping himself and the coffee upright it didn't give his mind the chance to flip out on him again? Didn't know and didn't really care, he was just so relieved to have made it.

He hoped to god that sort of journey would never happen to him again, he didn't think his heart could take it.

He was still trembling as he made his way out with a tide of bodies and into the haloed light of the open air.

When he stopped to fumble for his cigarettes his hands were visibly shaking again. A fresh surge of hostile travellers barged and knocked their way past as he struggled to take the lid off of the coffee and light his smoke. He could have spilt the still scolding liquid everywhere.

He had to wonder again if these people would be so discourteous if they knew their behaviour could actually jeopardize the already flimsy resolve of their weary saviour? The man who was going to sacrifice everything for them.

Will suddenly thought he was sounding like Jesus. He had to smirk at that one as he pressed the lid of his coffee back into place.

Anyway, to be honest he wasn't sacrificing himself for any of those selfish bastards. He liked to think he was doing it for the only two things that really mattered, love and friendship. Not the broad notion of them, just those individuals for whom he felt such emotions.

The times he'd struggled with his own ideas of how to express the depth of feeling he had for Becks. Grant you, he was normally pissed when he went off on such musings, but it didn't matter, it was here now, the opportunity had knocked and there were few of his generation who had ever had the chance to be heroic and prove their love.

He would have to try to cling to those sentiments as some kind of consolation when the time came, but for now he was still too scared and too weak to gain any real comfort.

He was even having trouble persuading himself to finish the final part of his trek and actually enter the office. He was dreading it, so much so it was making him nauseous.

Fuck it! He'd have another cigarette first. It would calm him down he reasoned, but he knew he was only delaying the inevitable.

He couldn't have picked a worse place to light up either; standing outside the building this early in the morning when everyone was coming into work. He edged back and sat on the low wall that separated the bland evergreen plant life of the office gardens from the pathway.

It would have been nice to at least have had a few short drafts of the coffee while he smoked but he found it was still scolding hot once he'd carefully taken the lid back off and in frustration he poured it into the plants.

Then it suddenly occurred to him that he would have to keep a special eye out for the cabs as they turned the corner. Clive would usually be in by now, but bet your life today he'd be a little bit later for some unexplained reason and Will really didn't want Clive to find him outside like that, just sitting on a wall and if nothing else Clive hated smoking.

It wouldn't give the impression he was hoping for... enthusiastic, enterprising, up for any fresh challenge!

There was no way Clive would knowingly saddle anyone on his level in the group with a loser, which Will had little doubt was Clive's view of him at present so he needed every other single little thing to be positive or at least not count as a negative. He was even going to wash his hands to get rid of the aroma of nicotine before he made the visit to Clive's office and make sure he hitched his tie knot right to the top of his shirt. He'd make sure he could recite the latest spot prices should it come up in conversation too. Suck up properly to the sour old bastard.

First things first though, it would help enormously if he could stop his hands from shaking.

'Pull yourself together.' He muttered, loud enough to startle a woman about to enter the revolving doors of the building.

Will watched her through the smoked glass until she disappeared from sight. He was relieved to see she didn't work for his organisation.

He extinguished the cigarette and made his own way through the doors towards the lifts.

Were the receptionists looking at him strangely? It felt like they were and he could feel their eyes boring a hole into the back of his head as he walked through the wide reception area.

He faced himself in the lift's mirror and inspected his reflection with disdain.

He appeared quite dishevelled he decided and not the least bit suave. A long way from suave, in fact a fucking wreck really after that journey and he wreaked of smoke, not just his nicotine stained fingers but his clothes, his breath everything.

This really wasn't what he had planned and in truth he just felt peculiar, so much so he just couldn't envisage snapping out of it well enough to confront Clive.

Sort yourself out Will! He urged himself silently in the moment before stepping out of the lift at his floor.

Perhaps it had worked because once he'd sneaked to his desk and sat down he felt a whole lot better. The air conditioning seemed to help. Will found the chill quite soothing, it seemed to relax him a little.

He felt if everyone left him alone he might just be alright. Calm down for a while then go and get himself straightened out in the gents. Who knew he might even be able to talk himself into knocking on Clive's door after all?

Will took a tentative peak over the end partition but Clive wasn't in his office yet which probably meant he was travelling as he was very rarely as late as this.

He couldn't say he was disappointed even if it was just postponing things.

Now that he had some breathing space he could for the first time since he'd left the office on the Friday before turn his thoughts to the job he was actually employed to do.

It was deadline day to close out the July white position on the exchange which suited him perfectly. It meant he'd be so busy his mind wouldn't be elsewhere thinking about Clive, or worse, thinking about Becks... his beautiful Becks.

There were other things to do as well, the real bread and butter stuff and he could get on and do them mechanically without much disturbance.

Only Alan and Ken were on the main desk and they were both absorbed in something and appeared nicely subdued.

Will began to view his present circumstances as a real slice of luck, not that he didn't feel he was due some, none the less he was thankful.

With Clive away, he had the time to clue up on the energy markets using the firm's portholes when he was finished doing the sugar stuff and if the boys were busy they wouldn't be asking questions as to why he was doing it.

The best bit of luck though was he could be prepared for tomorrow's journey in and arrive at the office in good shape. He was going to leave home at the crack of dawn and if he started feeling weird again he could simply get off, calm down and get the next train without making himself late.

He even contemplated going to buy a new suit at lunchtime as he didn't have any fresh ones in his wardrobe and he might even go for something a bit more sombre than usual, something more to Clive's liking. He would need to find out when the old bastard was back so he could be wearing it.

Now he was actually feeling positive for a change and he was determined to stay that way.

He'd close out the position, then sort out the physical delivery of a sale Peta had been dealing with and after, instead of revaluing the stock he was going to have a good read on Bloomberg and Reuters and see what was going on in the world of Energy.

****

For the first couple of hours things couldn't have gone better. The office had been so quiet that Will had barely looked up from his screens. He'd flattened most of the position and he'd even managed to track Peta down in the Paris office to consult him on the finer aspects of his physical deal.

However, at 11:21 a.m. the fire alarms went off. Will remembered specifically looking at the time in the corner of his Reuters screen when the alarm started. There was nothing unusual in this. The roasting machine emissions from the Coffee Department were always setting off the alarms or a car engine would overheat in the car park under the building.

Will would usually relish the opportunity to stretch his legs and smoke a cigarette while having a flirt with the girls from the accounts department as the fire warden recorded their attendance. But today the timing of the alarm couldn't have been worse for him.

There was barely an hour for him to arrange for Peta's warrants to be moved and there were positions to be rolled before twelve.

Anxiety hit him as soon as he set foot into the open air. His legs were shaking again and he was gasping a little for breath. Under normal circumstances he would have been stressed by the situation but he would just have ridden it out, chain smoked perhaps, cursed impatiently as he waited for the fire service to arrive and go about their business, but he would have stayed in control.

Today however, it was all too much for him; all of a sudden he was hit with an almighty sense of dread and found himself clinging to the glass façade of the building for dear life. He was falling apart, his legs had started shaking so much it impaired his ability to walk properly and that realisation absolutely terrified him with all of those people around him and it just left him *gasping* for breath and his chest became so constricted it felt like he needed to consciously force the air inside him, quicker and quicker just to catch his breath.

Someone grabbed his elbow from behind just when it seemed he was certain to stumble.

'Easy tiger!' Alan said jovially.

Will rolled his eyes barely able to focus let alone speak and he was feeling light headed now. Alan kept his hand where it was to steady him.

'What's up pal?' He asked with unease.

Will had to concentrate to get his dry tongue working.

'I'm just tense.' He gasped finally.

'Well you look it.' Alan observed.

Will struggled for a time to explain the immediate thing that was vexing him.

'Just calm down,' Alan advised in that soothing tone he had, 'nothing you can do is there? It's not your fault is it?'

Will grimaced as Alan put a comforting arm around him, more to save him from tears than embarrassment.

'Go on, have one of your cancer sticks and relax with yer old mate Al.' His friend said calmly.

Soon the pair watched the fire engine reverse out of the goods entrance and disappear around the corner.

They were left to trundle back up to their floor through the fire escape along with everyone else who couldn't wait in the queue for the lifts to operate again.

It was so frustrating for Will to be caught behind so many others on the slow assent that he could feel himself growing anxious all over again.

Yet there was still enough time for Will to finish the business with the exchange and having finally arrived on their floor he moved swiftly past Alan and onto the desk to call them.

The line was dead. Will reached over onto the dealer board and grabbed another receiver, dead as well. Exasperated he called out across the floor.

'Anyone's phone work? Anyone got a line!'

People began to pick up their receivers in search of a dialling tone but the whole floor was out. The alarm had taken down the main frame putting a temporary halt to all electrical functions other than the independent lighting.

'No screens no nothing!' Alan ranted. 'Where the fucks the IT guys?'

Will sat down at his desk clutching his head in despair, his breathing had become erratic again and he wished to god he had something neat to drink.

The minutes raced past until he knew he'd missed his deadline with the exchange. He was visibly shaking again and his heart was pounding so fast it actually felt like it might explode or just simply stop altogether. Then the power came back on and all of the telephones began to ring in abrupt unison.

Alan and Ken immediately began to try and placate them but the noise of it all began to jink hard on Will.

Peta came on the line to get an update on his deal and Ken swiftly passed the call over to Will.

He was quite churlish in response to the news that it hadn't been done and Will had to shout him down so he could explain he needed to get off the line to speak to the exchange for any chance of rectifying the problem.

When he did finally manage to speak to his contact and explain the delay he was relieved to learn that he would, as a special favour to Will, extend the cut-off for a few minutes.

It was enough time to enter the trade on the platform and send the fax releasing Peta's sugar. It was even enough time to receive the call explaining that he'd failed to sign the faxed document. However, it wasn't long enough to resend the fax before the main frame went down again.

Will remembered the next incident as if he'd only dreamt it, almost as though he was simply a bystander watching it all in slow motion.

It had taken some strength to rip the fax machine from its cord and launch it as far as he had across the office, Alan and Ken couldn't dispute that, neither could anyone else who happened to be watching. By the time he was kicking the thing, just before he stumbled over, everyone had an opinion. He'd captured everyone's attention with the screech he'd made.

Alan had been the one to pull him up and put him in a chair before escorting him into the lift and then into a taxi. Will had seen everyone divert their attention to their screens in solemn silence as he and Alan shuffled past.

Then as soon as they'd gone the IT boys began picking up the scatterings of the fax machine.

Clive tried to clear his throat, tried again and blew his nose ferociously but to little effect. It seemed he could never quite shift the catarrh in the warm weather. Still, there was some comfort in making the attempt to unclog the tubes without being growled at as he would be at home.

He was just returning his handkerchief to its jacket pocket when Sheila ducked her head through the door, beaming that inane grin of hers.

'Morning Clive.' She trilled through an implausible amount of teeth.

'Good trip?' She asked without waiting for a response.

'Will Shepherd is on his way up and I'm just off to collect him from the lift... would you like me to put him in my office and have you join us later or would you rather I brought him straight here?'

Clive considered the question solemnly.

'I think we'd better get the main task out of the way first and then perhaps you can take him off to your office to go over the finer details. I don't really want to get bogged down with all the finances etcetera... if that's ok with you?'

Had to be of course, now that the woman finally had something to do which fit her job description as opposed to god knows whatever else they were paying her for.

Clive would have liked to have got himself a cup of tea before the meeting but he didn't want to abandon the formality of the occasion. He just knew if he were to prance off to the kitchen now the stupid woman would soon follow, no doubt with Shepherd in tow and they would find themselves prattling on about the coming weekend with all and sundry and any sort of formality befitting the occasion would be gone.

No question then, the tea would have to wait. Nevertheless, Clive could quite happily defer a cup of tea in exchange for getting a dead weight like Shepherd off of the desk.

With that in mind he took a quick glance around the trading desk and spotted Kenneth on one side and the new Chinese chap on the other. It would do them good to witness a little taste of his retribution. He suddenly noticed Alan there too on the other side of the desk-divider, slumped low down in his chair like a slob, no doubt stuffing his fat face as usual. Well, the next little show might just make him get his size tens down from the desk and actually show a bit of commitment for a change.

Will inspected himself in the mirror as the lift glided upward. He decided he looked fully presentable for a change.

It appeared to him he was turned out well enough to be attending a job interview which under the circumstances seemed fairly apt.

It was a strange enough feeling having to register himself at reception but now he was going to be met in the foyer by HR as though it really were an interview.

To be honest Will suspected something like this was on the cards since the Tuesday evening when Sheila had called him at home. She wanted to check he was okay she'd said. Everyone was a little bit concerned apparently, even Clive. Of course he was; so concerned in fact that he'd even suggested to Sheila that it would be better if Will didn't return to the office until Friday. It would give him the chance to unwind a bit after his *turn* was how she'd put it and besides Clive wouldn't be back in the office until Friday.

Will couldn't quite see what relevance it was for Clive to have to be in the office when he went back until Sheila managed to work into the conversation that Will's fob thingy might not be working on his return as someone from the IT Dept. had disabled it by mistake.

Not very subtle, in fact pretty ridiculous to say something like that considering if you lost your key fob or had some other technical problem with it that stopped you getting through the doors you could just phone the help desk and you'd be sorted in minutes.

It was clear to him then that Clive was going to give him the mother of all dressing downs and what was to say he wouldn't just stop at threats this time and actually give him his notice? Wasn't really the company's way strictly speaking but then as far as Will was concerned there hadn't been any other occasion when someone had launched a fax machine across the office. He just had to hope and pray Clive wouldn't take it that far.

'You'll be a legend if he lets yer get away with this one.' Alan had commented when they'd spoken on Tuesday morning.

But Alan was worried about him Will could sense it, although Will had batted his concerns away. Just felt he had to appear strong if nothing else. If Alan could have actually seen him that day he got home well...

He'd been too scared to even drink then; just sitting on the sofa quaking.

He even took the advice Al gave him as he was putting him into the cab that took him home and had gone to see the doctor. Had to go as an emergency and wait around to the very end of surgery hours until all the appointments were finished but he had to say it was the best thing he'd ever done.

He really was an emergency anyway, in truth, couldn't sit still, couldn't focus on anything, just a bag of nerves slipping in and out of the surgery to have a smoke which had really pissed off the receptionist.

The doctor was great. Will told him he couldn't sleep but obviously didn't tell him why and said he was really stressed out at work and even stressed just getting to work and while he was saying it his voice cracked a little.

So, the doctor signed him off then and there for four weeks, not that Will had any intention of staying off of work for a second longer than need be. He really wanted to get straight back and get his future resolved and get his plan working. Didn't know how he was going to find the strength to do that to be honest but then the Doctor wrote out the prescription for the Diazepam. They were tranquilizers and what a godsend they were. He'd taken more than he should that first night but boy did he sleep.

He found if he kept himself properly doped up he could even get on the pc and do a bit of research about what went on in the oil world and what sort of hedging went on against the physical products. All seemed straight forward enough. It was just the guys doing the physical itself that needed the real brains. He shouldn't have wondered they needed to have a chemistry degree it all looked so complicated. Still no one would expect him to get his head around that stuff he was sure.

He was confident enough he could do what he needed to do which would be enough to make a difference to the markets if he ever got the opportunity.

He had lost all of his appetite and could barely eat anything, which he thought must have had something to do with the tranquilizers, but in the big scheme of things considering how he had felt before he'd taken them, not being able to eat was a good trade off and he should be thankful.

In all honesty it was a stone fucking miracle he'd managed to come back to work at all and was actually going up in the lift.

Somehow those drugs were keeping him in control and had given him a chance to make amends and try again with his plan.

Now Will actually felt ready, or at least as ready as he was ever going to be. He just had to keep himself together and if he was going to start shaking he'd have to do what he'd practiced and squeeze his hands tightly together and dig a nail into the skin, the sort of distraction they used to use in the old war films when they were getting tortured and he had an extra little pill in his jacket pocket just in case.

Whatever it took was worth it. To make this meeting with Clive go right was easily the most important thing he had ever done in his life. Complete subjugation was the order of the day he'd decided. Let Clive have his rant then Will would do all the apologies and grovelling he could muster until Clive was satisfied he'd destroyed him enough and then Will would give him the out and introduce the idea of a transfer to the Energy division. Will was sure that Clive would have worked himself into such a stew by then he'd simply jump at the chance to move him on and agree to the idea immediately.

It was a sure thing, unquestionable in Will's mind. For all of Clive's ranting no one got the push properly, Alan had said it, everyone knew it, you just got moved on to something shit that they knew you wouldn't want to do in the hope you'd be pissed off enough to go away by yourself and for it to be Will making the suggestion it was going to be alright. Well it had to be.

He *had* to get exposure to the oil markets. It was easily the best and probably the only opportunity he would get to be in any sort of position to transform or manipulate forthcoming events.

Will reached his floor and the doors were opening and suddenly out of nowhere he had that familiar feeling of utter panic, but he was determined to stay calm. Go on Billy boy, he pleaded with his reflection... please stay calm, and just for now he was going to hold back on slipping the hidden pill into his mouth.

Sheila was waiting in the lobby with a grin as radiant as it was insincere.

'How are you?' She cooed. 'How was the journey in?'

'Fine.' He told her. He couldn't mention that without the drugs he felt like he might die every time he stepped onto a train and he definitely wouldn't mention that lately it felt like the clouds were poised to suffocate him like a scattering of giant pillows. She wouldn't be sympathetic and she would never be on his side.

He just had to act normal and take deep breaths. Stay calm. Sheila used her key fob and held the door for him as he entered giving him the full visitors' treatment.

Will took a fleeting look over at the trading desk. Alan and Ken were in their usual places and even Peta was there with some other dude.

He raised a hand meekly to return their sombre greetings and followed Sheila's large behind along the familiar gangway while she expertly chirped away about nothing in particular to fill the empty time.

The atmosphere was many degrees frostier once the two of them had entered Clive's office.

Clive had just about managed to mutter some sort of greeting before slapping down the correspondence he was pretending to read onto his desk and gesturing to Sheila to close the door.

'Have a seat.' He ordered, ushering them both abruptly into the chairs opposite him with his hand.

Sheila had finally put away her absurd grin.

'Okay, Will', Clive began. 'I can see very little point in beating about the bush. We all know why you're here and I just have to say you can consider yourself extremely fortunate that I wasn't around to witness your actions myself as I don't feel we'd even have gone so far as to arrange this meeting if I had.'

Clive paused there for the moment to let the full weight of his rhetoric be absorbed.

'From what I can gather from those unfortunate enough to have been present, your actions were totally unacceptable within the working practices of this company and will not be tolerated from anyone regardless of their position, length of service or any other factor you may wish to put forward.'

'I totally agree.' Will managed to concur in the moment Clive took to gather his thoughts in order to proceed.

'Yes, well,' Clive affirmed, 'I'm glad you feel some remorse for your actions which I presume means you'll fully understand the decision I've had to make?'

Will stared at his employer perplexed.

'What are you suggesting?' He asked meekly.

'What I'm suggesting Will is you discontinue working here.'

Will felt suddenly dazed.

'Now I'm sure you're aware your performance over a prolonged period of time has been open to serious question, but up until now I've been willing to reflect on your earlier endeavours and given you the benefit of the doubt. Unfortunately, the conduct shown last Monday was really the last straw!'

'But...' Will began but had been so taken aback he was struggling to find the right words that could turn the conversation around to how he'd imagined it unfolding.

'Please let me join Energy!' Was all he managed to blurt out just a moment before Clive was poised to continue and now he was sure the sudden outburst had ruined the considered argument he had practised and refined over and over in his head for days.

'Energy?' Clive asked in astonishment.

'Well the Energy desk are recruiting at the moment.' Sheila chipped in.

Clive gave her a scornful look.

'Well I hardly think a move to Energy is an option,' he stated firmly, 'given that we're terminating his contract on the grounds of misconduct Sheila! For heaven's sake woman!'

Will could have seen her shrink back into her chair then but he was desperately preoccupied on coaxing something from his mind that could save his situation.

'I just feel a fresh start would work for me.' Will persisted. 'Well I'm very sorry, I'm just not willing to follow this path any further.' Clive said sternly as he sunk both palms of his hands down into the leather of his desk in a gesture affirming his stance.

Still Will persevered. He had no choice. He was even prepared to beg.

'Please Clive,' he pleaded, 'I'm begging you to give me one last chance.'

'Oh, for fucks sake!' Clive gasped, slamming his palms down so loudly this time the clap could be heard outside his door and right across the trading desks.

'There will be a very considerate annuity package.' Sheila volunteered quickly despite some apprehension.

'But I need to work for *Energy*!' Will snapped, exposing the size of his desperation with the tone.

Now with patience exhausted Clive pushed himself up from the chair he had only just sunk into, his hands aloft like shields against any further remonstrations.

'I'm sorry but that really is enough.' He said firmly. 'I've made my decision and I fully intend to stick to it.'

Will matching Clive's tenacity began again but this time Clive interrupted him with a resonance louder and even more forceful than before.

'I'm afraid this discussion is over Will!' He asserted. 'I'm as sorry as I am surprised you've taken the news so badly but I really must put an end to this and get on... Sheila here will be happy to work through the details of the annulment with you in her office.'

After a very brief relapse Sheila recovered from her own shock on how volatile the meeting had turned and got to her feet and was mumbling her compliance when the full extent of Will's anguish engulfed him then unleashed itself on the room.

He later remembered it had felt as if he were falling, but he hadn't moved, couldn't move in fact. His legs had seemed to vibrate and both his thoughts and the words he needed to deliver seemed to swim around him until he was gasping for breath and then he was howling. In his own head or loudly enough for the whole world to hear he really couldn't tell nor could he see Sheila's concerned face through his tears, though he did catch her soothing words while she patted his shoulder.

'You'll receive a good package.' She'd said. 'A very good reference!'

And when neither of those had placated him there was mention of further financial aid if needed, though by then he was on his knees with Sheila probably on hers beside him.

Will didn't remember much of the commotion that followed. Hadn't seen Clive flustered with equal measures of alarm and disgust as he watched Alan's face, who had suddenly appeared, glow with such barely concealed rage at Clive while simultaneously trying to comfort his friend.

A lady from the Finance Department had been dragged along by Sheila to administer her own crude version of first aid, lying him down, covering him up.

Then he remembered shaking almost in spasms and feeling as though he might be having a proper fit and then the ambulance crew had got there.

They'd quickly calmed him down then, familiar and friendly yet business like as though, Will was sure, they'd seen the same sort of thing millions of times before, making him feel ridiculous. They made the whole episode appear as it was, hysterical and trivial.

The mood suddenly changed from alarm to bemusement and Will's own slant changed from abject terror to a vague sense of embarrassment and he wasn't quite sure which of the two he preferred as they took him down to the ambulance in a wheelchair with a blanket wrapped around him and Sheila by his side.

He was beginning to feel numb by then he supposed, for want of a better expression. Numb, exhausted and beaten. But just then, just for that brief period when they drove him to the hospital wrapped in that blanket, he didn't care about anything at all and it had felt so bloody liberating.

'What's the matter?' A curt young paramedic asked him as he was wheeled through the A&E emergency doors at St Thomas's.

Was Will crying? He couldn't remember.

'Are you actually ill?' The young man asked.

'I don't know.' Will answered feebly.

'Well look around you,' the paramedic continued, 'we're very busy and unless you can explain why you're here I'm gonna ask you to get out of that chair and go home.'

'Now hang on!' Sheila objected. 'You can see he's clearly unwell!'

'Fine!' Said the young man. 'Tell him to get out of the wheelchair and go and sit with everyone else in the waiting room and wait his turn!'

Sheila duly obliged, helping Will out of his seat as he tested the strength of his shaking legs.

They shuffled out of the swing doors and over to some plastic seats that were bound rigidly together at the far end of the waiting room.

'There.' Sheila said as he lowered himself into a seat.

'I'm going to the reception to make sure you've been booked in.'

Will watched her go, her large arse once again bounding purposely away.

There was a queue at the reception so Will was left alone. He looked around the room which was half full... well not quite half but then it was just a Friday afternoon.

Some visible injuries; A young boy still in his football kit clutching his shin and clearly in pain, a very old man in a wheelchair seemingly disorientated, having a cut above his eye patted and squeezed by another slightly younger looking man with a handkerchief, his son perhaps?

There didn't seem anything wrong with anyone else, they were just sitting there. Most of them with companions but it wasn't particularly easy to see which was the patient and which the companion.

What about him then? If there was anyone in the room faking, it had to be him. He just wanted to go home, get properly pissed and take a handful of the pills. His life had reached that true point now of worthlessness. Everything about him.

When Sheila finally returned she sat beside him and patted his thigh and gave him another of her standard smiles.

'It's going to be a bit of a wait but you're on the list and we'll just have to wait and see.'

'You shouldn't wait.' Will said.

'We'll see.' She said.

'There's nothing wrong with me really... you heard what that doctor said.'

'Well actually I don't even think he was a doctor and either way the prognosis seemed a little rash to me dear.'

'Just go Sheila, you've been very kind but I don't want you hanging around here... you might catch something.' He said glumly.

'It's fine.' She said patting his knee again.

They waited endlessly then. The silence broken only by Sheila's maternal instincts ensuring he was comfortable or wasn't thirsty.

It came to the point when Will became very aware of the time, it now being very close to the end of office hours.

He was just about to try to persuade Sheila to leave again when before he could speak there was someone familiar who had just entered the room.

Her hair swaying to and fro as she hurriedly looked around, concern etched all over her face, but when she spotted him that immaculate grin he loved so much lit the room and Will's weary heart.

She literally ran over to him and Will suddenly broke down in tears and used all of the energy he could to stand to greet her and they clasped their bodies together and both were crying with what looked to Sheila... pure joy.

'I didn't expect that.' Will said lifting his head from between his knees.

'What?' Becky asked.

'Sheila staying all that time.'

'I know, it was really good of her.'

'She's not like that at work you know… people think she's a bit of a joke.'

'Well there you are.' Becky remarked.

The doors swung open but it was just a porter lumbering through with a trolley.

'You can still go you know?' Will said.

'Look, just fuck off!' She gasped.

'Good.' He croaked and then he was sobbing uncontrollably again.

Becky slid closer to him and began gently stroking his neck and shoulders.

'I'm not going anywhere Will.' She whispered. 'You understand me don't you?'

Will nodded his head.

'I'm never going away again.'

'But I'm just a worthless piece of shit!' He blubbed through his snot and tears while a string of mucus bounced between his lips.

'You're not Will, you're not!' She said forcefully as she smoothed the worst of the mess from his face with the palm of her hand.

'It's just like the real doctor said, you're ill that's all, you're ill and I'm going to look after you and you're going to get better.'

Becky looked down at her watch. It was ridiculous now, they'd already waited twenty minutes longer for the cab than they were supposed to. She was just praying the driver hadn't got lost like she had when she'd arrived with so many entrances and exits in the hospital. The last thing she wanted was the casualties from the pubs to start turning up drunk, not with Will crying and everything, what a target he'd be.

She took a deep breath and raised herself from her seat trying to decide if it was worth the grief of going to phone the taxi firm again and leaving Will alone for however long.

She just wished the doctor had given Will something to calm him down. It was all very well saying the prescription he'd been given by his GP wasn't right for him but he could have at least found some different ones to take that were.

He'd been very kind and everything but all the doctor had actually done after all of that waiting was to say he was suffering from anxiety. He said with all the recent turmoil in his life it was probably a blessing in disguise to have had such a stressful job taken away from him. Becky agreed with that of course and that Will needed to get some real rest but then he'd just advised him to go and see his GP again. The same man who had prescribed inappropriate tablets and had just sent him away. Where was the sense in that?

Sheila had been brilliant then. She thought going back to the GP was a ridiculous idea too and then she said, because Will had had his *turn* before any of the paperwork had been signed, technically he was still an employee which meant he was still covered by the company's medical insurance.

She said Will only needed to go back to the GP to get a referral to a specialist and she would make sure the company honoured whatever the cost of the treatment was going to be.

She really didn't have to do that and Will had been worried that she might actually get into trouble with Clive for suggesting it but Sheila was insistent.

'I'm the HR manager Will,' she said bluntly, 'and if Clive wants to kick up a stink we shall have to see what our Chairman has to say.'

Thank god.

'Taxi for Rebecca Shepherd.' Someone mumbled into the tannoy system.

Becky looked over to the reception area but didn't see anyone likely to be driving a cab in the queue, then over by the exit she saw an old West Indian guy jingle some keys in his enormous hands.

'Taxi for Rebecca Shepherd.' The tannoy sounded again.

'It's us!' She called raising an arm.

He disappeared instantly through the doors with his keys still jingling.

He couldn't just fuck off like that she seethed, he had to wait. It was going to take Will ages to walk outside and she didn't have a clue where to go.

She'd got Will to his feet easily enough but it really had taken ages to get as far as the door and now the driver had come back looking all impatient.

'Yes, well my husband's not very well if you hadn't noticed!' She fumed.

Idiot, Becky thought and decided she was going to take a leaf out of Will's book and make a point of holding back a tip.

James woke up face down in his clothes again.

Some fucker must have literally smashed the front door shut. His tongue was cloying for moisture and he hung his hand carefully over the bed to feel his way around the floor blindly searching for the plastic bottle that had been filled and refilled with the water from the bathroom tap, moving slowly so as not to place his fingers over the edges of his recently acquired piss-pot.

It wasn't in reach but he couldn't quite summon the courage to pull himself up for a proper look around. Not just yet.

With any luck his thirst could be abated for a while, long enough for him to fall back into another dead sleep, so yesterday, in fact all of his recent life, could be forgotten again if only for a few short hours.

Heaven only knew what Brian thought of him after the previous evening's carry on?

He had knocked on his door already much the worse for wear practically begging a drink and some company but then had the audacity to accuse the poor man of unwanted interference and to mind his own business simply because he had given, what on the face of it, was thoughtful and sound advice on how to handle the crisis James was facing and a perfectly admissible answer on how to regain access to his sons.

'Take 'er through the fackin courts.' Brian had suggested, but James had immediately baulked at the suggestion knowing what a fierce adversary Deborah could be.

'Then at the least threaten 'er with it!' Brian had pleaded quite venomously.

James had had no intention of doing that either but now the seed had been sown in his mind and all it took was for the bitch to rile him once more the very next time they spoke.

So then, during the verbal sparring match they conducted daily over the phone at his expense, she had continued with the notion that he had to hand her cash for the right to visit his own children.

'You know damn well I have every right to see the boys regardless of my financial circumstances and if you continue to obstruct me you know what I can do don't you?'

'Excuse me? She exclaimed.

'Now let's not play games Deborah. You know just as well as I do that I could use the legal route and gain access through the courts.'

He had worked himself up into quite a stupor by this stage and when her immediate response was simply to smirk down the line he lost control completely.

'So be it!' He'd bellowed at her, feeling every bit as ridiculous as he no doubt sounded. 'I shall visit the Citizens' Advice office this afternoon!'

He was certain she would hang up the phone at that point as she had a habit of doing once the argument had become unsatisfactory to her, but he was astonished to find she was still there. In hindsight James concurred that she had been waiting very patiently for such an opportunity to present itself and he wouldn't have been the least bit surprised if the course of the exchange that followed hadn't been both schemed and rehearsed vigorously in her head.

'Well there isn't any judge female or male who'd think you were fit to be a father.'

'Oh yes,' he replied, 'and on what grounds?'

'You know what grounds you sad pervert.'

'You silly bitch.' He'd scoffed, certain the receiver would be slammed down this time, but again he was mistaken.

'Do you honestly believe any court in the land would be so offended by something as innocent... and may I remind you, completely legal...'

'Innocent?' She interrupted.

'Yes Deborah, innocent.'

But he had tried to persuade her so many times before he knew it was useless.

'Fine!' She'd shrieked and then, and this is what he was sure she had been building up to all along, she landed the killer blow.

'Let's see what the boys think shall we?'

James had immediately hung his head in abject defeat. He fought so hard then to keep his response even toned and his voice unwavering.

'Not even you would stoop so low as to damage our children's happiness any further.' He reasoned.

'But if it's all so innocent you ain't got anything to worry about have you?'

James physically buckled then in the cramped space of the telephone booth, stooping now and barely holding his thoughts together, he grasped onto the phone casing to prevent him from collapsing altogether down onto the squalid square of ground where the filth had been allowed to mass and congeal at the corners unshifted by the rivers of piss that had inadvertently tried to displace it over the years.

'Understood.' He whispered.

'Okay then, speak to you later.' And she was back to that aloof manner he now despised.

Now the receiver did go down and without any malice, just a victorious click.

He had been completely overthrown again.

James clambered back straight onto his feet but he couldn't think what to do next. The angst rising up inside him left him in such a whirl of desperation for an outlet that he did what he supposed most men might do in his situation. Foolishly, typically, he headed for the nearest pub.

In all honesty it would have been fine if it had ended there. He would easily have forgiven himself if he had merely spent a few hours drowning his sorrows but the pub he had gone to was virtually empty and he sat for a while in its saloon bar drinking at a conspicuous speed for the surroundings, his rage undiminished and it was then he had resolved to catch a bus and head to his old stomping ground in Romford and to the *Parvs* bar for the Stella beer and some lively distraction.

James groaned into his pillow. These reflections weren't helping him ease towards sleep at all.

For one thing he had suddenly remembered he had spent nearly every spare bit of cash he had in the world, every pound if not every penny and now he wasn't quite sure what he was going to do for food for the remainder of the week. Hopefully he could scrape together enough coins to buy a loaf of bread which he would have to eek out until the Giro arrived.

He wouldn't dare allow himself any sympathy because he'd been so bloody reckless. *Parvs* had done the trick early on but he had happily stayed and wallowed in the drink and the endless fascination of that environment.

You certainly got to hear all manner of extraordinary conversations in that type of place James had noticed.

There were two ladies of a certain age leaning with their backs to the bar as he entered and waited to be served. Both of them dressed in sportswear although it was clear neither participated in any sort of sporting activity judging by their figures and neither seemed in any hurry to take up anything physical considering they were both puffing furiously on cigarettes.

'If 'e ain't beating me up 'is crying and if 'e ain't crying 'is beating me up.' One of them had explained to her friend. Tragic really James surmised.

Later there was a young mother, also in sportswear, though far more appropriate looking, elegant and athletic, who wandered into the bar clutching a small child in pigtails by the hand, seeking out what must have been her partner at the far end of the bar and when they came together there was very little dialogue but plenty of kisses for both mother and child. A brief but very affectionate coming together until the young lady headed back toward the door. Her little girl, he could see now wearing her ballet costume, so pink and pretty. Trying her very best to pirouette as they walked and simply skipping when she couldn't, bobbing her head happily and seeming utterly content within the world she occupied.

It wasn't so long ago that James would have been horrified to see a child paraded through such a place and no doubt familiar with the surroundings, but who was he to judge now? Were his children as happy as that little girl? Somehow, he doubted it, could they ever be truly happy again? Sadly, he doubted that too and the idea would crush him completely if he allowed himself to dwell on it for too long.

Really, he should have left the bar soon after the girl and her mother had gone as he had reached that nice point of finally being subdued and just tipsy enough to make the trek home in a sensible fashion before insouciance set in. Instead he persuaded himself to have that fabled 'one for the road' and found himself several hours later still at his little table like so many of the other older men sitting alone in silence while the guttural laughter of those more fortunate who stood in groups washed over them.

There was a time when he could regard himself as a mere observer and return to his normal life but the sad truth was he knew he was one of them now. Middle aged, unemployed, practically homeless, virtually penniless and if he were brutally honest would have to say bordering on an alcoholic, or at least would be if he could afford it.

No way back to Deborah and the boys and all because of that misunderstanding. Just for the lack of communication that the British seemed to suffer from as they failed miserably to express their desires and needs with regard to anything coital.

James wondered what Deborah had done with the magazine. He hoped to god she was vigilant enough to hide it well from the boys. It would be shocking for them to come across something as rude in the sanctity of their own home regardless of whether they reached the page that had the photo on it.

Would they identify their own father anyway? Deborah seemed to have trouble recognizing him even when he'd pointed it out to her.

All of the pictures had been a disappointment to him when he had finally summoned the courage to retrieve them from the chemist. The one he had sent to the magazine was only the best of a bad bunch, the image reflected from the mirror on the wardrobe door. He had polished the mirror scrupulously but the effect was still dusty and slightly blurred.

It was strange how he still managed to giggle at the memory of playing with himself to give the best effect without being too stiff. They couldn't publish it if you were erect.

The horror on Deborah's face when she read the blurb that accompanied it.

'A playmate for us both please.' Just as she herself had intimated and why was it so different to move what could still remain a fantasy onto the next level?

James didn't want to be drawn back into that debate which had gone on endlessly in his head.

He should really try hard to sleep now and in all honesty there was very little reason to wake again.

Becky's dad drove off to park the car leaving the three of them by the entrance.

Thank god for her mum and dad's help she thought. God only knew how she would have coped without it.

That Sheila from his work had been so brilliant as well. Somehow, she'd bypassed Will's doctor completely and gone straight to BUPA and set up an appointment with this psychiatrist fella.

He was meant to be very good according to Sheila and Becky couldn't thank her enough and she was so incredibly touched by her kindness. In fact, she couldn't help get a little bit emotional when she was on the phone to her and it sounded like Sheila had got a little choked up as well. It was nice really, even if it was embarrassing. At least it proved she was grateful.

'Let's go in,' her mum said, 'your dad'll find us.'

The place wasn't very big anyway, just one square room with a reception area at the far end and a scattering of nice armchairs and coffee tables. The armchairs mostly filled with old people, some of them chatting quietly or sipping their complimentary teas and coffees from a fancy drinks dispenser in one of the corners.

They could almost be in an airport lounge Becky thought, if the signs they had up were directing you to the duty-free rather than x-ray or cardiology.

Definitely hadn't been like that at Saint Thomas's.

It hadn't been that difficult getting Will through the doors either as they just swished open when they got close to them and only closed again when they were safely through, her on one side and her mum on the other.

They managed to put Will down in one of the upright chairs opposite the reception desk.

He was in such a bloody state and it frightened her so much, shaking, welling-up all the time, not really divulging anything about why.

'We've got an appointment with Doctor Julian Baker.' She said to the first receptionist as soon as she'd come off the phone and looked up at her.

'It's for William Shepherd.'

'Let's see then.' The receptionist said in hushed tones before engaging the p.c. on the desk before her.

'Yes, that's fine... do take a seat.' She said smiling but no sooner had Becky sat down than this Doctor Baker appeared from behind a petition and called out Will's name.

'William Shepherd.' His deep voice resounded throughout the room.

By the look of him he wasn't what Becky had expected. She'd imagined someone in a tie and a white coat with a collection of pens in his breast pocket or if he didn't look like that she thought he might be someone in a tweed jacket with thick rimmed glasses and a great unruly beard. This guy didn't fit either bill. He looked more like a porter, black trousers, plain open shirt and what looked like some kind of hiking boots. His hair, what there was of it, was all a bit bedraggled too. Definitely wouldn't have thought a psychiatrist would look like that, but then she'd only really got the idea of what he was supposed to look like from the television, those shows where everyone looked glamorous like Dallas or Dynasty.

'You'll be fine.' Her mum was whispering into Will's ear as they both stood on either side of him to help him up.

'You'll get the right help here darling.' She said.

When they'd finally got him to the office through a labyrinth of corridors, with Doctor Baker holding each fire door patiently for them, they put Will in a chair nearest the desk and her mum went back to look for her dad.

They waited then for the doctor to arrange the blotter on his desk. He very neatly took a piece of paper from one of the trays and smoothed it carefully in front of him. Finally, he cleared his throat.

'Well William,' he said softly 'you're looking extremely anxious. Can you tell me how long you've been feeling this way?'

'Erm,' Will dithered, closing his eyes to consider the question.

'On and off for months really.' He managed to divulge, bowing his head like a bashful child as his cheeks flushed to betray his embarrassment.

'Have you been using any recreational drugs?'

'No.'

'Alcohol?'

'Yes.'

'A lot of alcohol?' The psychiatrist asked looking up from his notes and engaging Will eye to eye.

'I suppose so, yes.'

'And has this been the case for some time or would you say you've been using alcohol a little more recently to help you when you've been feeling anxious as a way of calming down?'

'Well, to tell you the truth,' Will said quietly as he passed a clammy hand over his brow, 'I've always liked a drink but I've been drinking a lot more since I've been you know... going doolally.'

'So, you're feeling unsettled all of the time regardless of any stimulants you may have been taking?'

'Feels like I'm losing the plot.' Will confessed.

'Okay, well yes.' The doctor said nodding his head appreciatively before returning to his notes.

'How's work been?' He asked after a short while.

'Stressful.' Will admitted.

'Since before or...'

'Both.'

'I see... and what is it you do?'

'Well I was a commodity trader until yesterday.'

'Oh, I see. So really quite stressful I should imagine?'

'It can be.'

'And have you been trading commodities long?'

'A few years.'

'A few years, okay.'

Will watched the doctor scribble furiously using all of the paper before him in a rolling text that he couldn't quite decipher from the angle he was sitting at then a second sheet was added to the blotter as before and smoothed down carefully.

'Any other concerns which may have caused you distress?'
'I don't know really.' He lied, but before Becks could interject he'd said it.

'My mum died in June.'
'Ah, well yes, that would certainly have had an effect.'
The doctor continued with his notes.
'Did you have a good relationship with your mother?'
'Yes.'

'Is your father alive?'
'No.'

'Ah I see. So, would you have regarded your relationship with your mother as close?'
'I suppose so... just like a normal mother and son.'
'Okay.' The doctor sighed looking up at Will for more eye contact.

'Would you say you had a happy childhood William?'
'Erm... it wasn't bad I suppose.'
The psychiatrist stared at him a little more intently.
'You seem a little undecided.'

'Well you know,' Will muttered 'a few bad episodes.'
'Such as?' The doctor asked before returning to the page with his pen.

'My father left when I was eight.'
'I see... and has he remained in contact?'
'No.'

'And you haven't seen him since he left?'
'No.'
'Do you remember feeling very upset about it?'
'Well yeah... of course.'
'And was your mother very upset?'
'I would have thought so.'
'But she didn't talk about it?'
'Not really. Not to me anyway.'
'And do you have brothers or sisters?'
'My brother died a few days before my dad left.'
Doctor Baker looked up from his writing and placed the lid back on the pen and placed it neatly onto the blotter.

'Okay.' He said with a deep sigh. 'Well I'm terribly sorry to hear that.' He added in earnest.

'And what age did you say you were William?'

'Eight.'

The doctor glanced over his paperwork and inserted a little note and the figure 8.

'And what age was your brother?'

'Eleven.'

'And what were the circumstances of his death?'

'A road accident.'

'Ahh...' The doctor sighed.

'Do you have any other brothers or sisters?'

'No.'

'I see.'

The doctor picked up his pen again and rested it on his chin, teasing the mound of skin with tiny taps as he drifted away for a while in quiet contemplation.

'I spoke very briefly to your GP,' he began on his return, 'and he informs me you have been having some trouble sleeping?'

'Yes.'

'And has this always been a problem?'

'Not really... only the last three or four months.'

'Soon after your mother passed away?'

'Yes, but that's not what's been stopping me sleeping. It's hard to explain. I've been having visions, you know... like nightmares but worse.'

'And does your mother appear in these nightmares?'

'No, not at all.'

Will cleared his throat and swallowed hard. The next revelation he was about to make was surely going to make him certifiable.

'The thing is doctor they're nothing like nightmares really,' he said with his voice quivering, 'they're visions. They're real visions.'

'Okay then,' the psychiatrist agreed quite unperturbed, 'visions.'

'And do you ever have these visions while you're awake?'

'No.'

'So only when you're completely asleep?'

'Yes, and I see your point, but trust me doctor these... what I experience is nothing like a dream or a nightmare!'

'How so?'

'Because they're so very real... it's like the guy I see in them... well I could almost reach out and touch him and he's always there telling me things, urging me to do things.'

Doctor Baker looked at him curiously.

'What sort of things does he tell you?'

'About the end of the world mostly... and about disasters that have happened before... all in London though, everything he's ever talked about happened in London.'

'Okay, very specific then?'

'Definitely.' Will affirmed, his voice gaining in excitement. 'The Blitz, the plague... you know, the Great Fire.'

'And these visions cause a lot of distress?'

'I suppose they must. I know they exasperate me and I try to respond to him but I just wake up.'

'Normally he calls out.' Becky quickly interrupted.

'I see.' The doctor said accepting the intrusion benignly.

'So, you're both missing out on sleep.'

'Not that I mind.' She moved to assure him.

'No, I'm sure.' He answered appreciatively.

'So, William,' he said returning to his patient, 'would you say you drink alcohol to help you to sleep, or rather, to help you remain asleep?'

'Yes,' Will agreed, 'but actually, it's more like I drink a lot to help me calm down, you know... to stop me getting so anxious.'

'Well I must say you seem extremely anxious now.'

Will looked at the psychiatrist resentfully, his jaw jutting outward which might even have been construed as petulance if it hadn't been for the fresh tears that had welled in his eyes.

'Yeah I am.' He confessed, feeling the trickles along the contours of his nose.

'And have you always been concerned by the threat of disaster?'

'No more than anyone else I wouldn't have thought.'

'So not inordinately?'

'No.' Will answered doubtfully.

'So not disproportionately?'

'No. Not before the visions.'

'Okay.'

'It's just that he wants me to stop another disaster.'

'He?'

'Yeah... this guy from my visions... his name's Thom.'

'And it's only him who pays you these visits?'

'Yes.'

'Does he remind you of anyone from your past?'

Will considered for a moment just to check his own thoughts again.

'No. No one I've known.'

'Not your father?'

'Definitely not and anyway he's miles... years older.'

'And you've never once heard him speak to you while you've been awake?'

'Not ever.'

The psychiatrist stared at Will intently for a while, deep in thought, then returned to his pen and resumed writing notes. After finishing a third page he unlocked a draw to his side and pulled out a prescription pad admonishing an explanation to the drugs he was about to prescribe as he filled the form.

'What I'm proposing to do William is offer medication which I'm confident will make you feel more at ease sooner rather than later. The first is a tranquilizer, quite unlike diazepam, which should help suppress the anxiety and at the very least give you a peaceful night's rest. The second will be a short course of neuroleptic drugs, which I am quite hopeful will improve your situation. Now you may feel alarmed while reading the leaflet which accompanies this second course of treatment as you'll come across such phrases as 'anti-psychotic' or 'schizophrenic' but please remember these are merely medical terms and must not in any way be confused with how they are conveyed in either film or television.'

'You do understand that don't you?' The psychiatrist asked and waited patiently for Will's nodded approval.

'Will I still be able to drink… you know… if it's getting too much?' Will asked.

'Well considering you've already been using alcohol and it doesn't seem to have been of any benefit I wouldn't recommend it.' The doctor said sternly.

'Fair enough.' Will had to concede fully aware of Becks shaking her head dismally out of the corner of his eye.

'There.' Doctor Baker said folding the prescription and passing it to Becky.

He pushed his chair away from his desk and swivelled around enabling him to rest his hands on his thighs.

'Now with the medication taken care of I'd like to discuss the idea of counselling with you.'

'Fine.' Will answered sceptically.

'I'm confident you may benefit considerably from it William and the chap I'd like to send you to is a close colleague of mine. He is a very well-regarded psychologist, his speciality being simply to listen to the issues which have been causing you distress and hopefully, with his careful guidance, help you understand and manage them better.'

'Are you willing to give him a try?'

'If you think it will help I suppose I ought to.' Will conceded.

'Well unfortunately I can't *guarantee* it will help but experience has shown me in cases such as yours there can be some real benefit to be had.'

'Well it can't do any harm can it?' Becky suggested placing a palm of her hand on Will's knee and stroking it gently.

'Although I must also warn you, some of our patients find the experience rather painful at times as well as uplifting.'

Will turned to his wife and smiled with the silent tears still rolling gently onto his cheeks.

'You ought to don't you think?' She asked and received the nod she was hoping for and now they were both in tears.

Becky's hand moved gently to squeeze Will's while Doctor Baker began writing something else on his own letter headed paper and having produced an envelope from another shelf handed this over to Becky as well.

'The chap's name I'm sending you to William is Frank O'Keefe and his secretary will no doubt be contacting you within the next day or two to book an appointment.

'I must advise you that the practice is a little off of the beaten track and not the easiest place to get to and although you may start feeling a little better after these new drugs take effect I wouldn't recommend attempting to drive for the time being so I'm afraid you're going to need some assistance in getting you there.'

'I hope that's going to be possible?' The doctor asked Becky.

'Yes, that's absolutely fine.' She assured him.

'Good. Very good and I shall arrange an appointment to see you again this time next week William.'

'Should however, you have any wish to speak with me before then, if perhaps you're having trouble coping, please don't hesitate to contact me.'

Doctor Baker smiled a very sincere smile for the both of them indicating the session had come to an end at which point Becky quickly stood up to help Will from his chair to which he politely declined.

The numbness in his legs had subsided somewhat and he was sure that if he moved slowly enough he could make it out through the door unaided.

Chapter 31 – Going to meet a new friend

The psychologist's office was miles from anywhere in a small alcove of rural Essex, wedged between the M11 and the M25, empty winding roads looking out onto flat churned fields. The green belt that made city dwellers feel free for a while, when as today, it was bathed in sunshine.

Will envisaged what a lovely drive it could have been if he weren't ill. How perfect it could be if he was well and he was at the wheel of a new Aston.

As it was Becks was in the driving seat looking tired and nervous. She never had liked driving when she didn't know where she was going and now she had the added worry of him like an invalid hunched beside her as well as having to find some remote place on time. He could see the tension etched on her face.

'You know I'm fine.' He kept telling her and he was. He'd taken an extra tranquillizer before they'd left. He'd been apprehensive before that. He'd been worried about the journey too, even a little frightened just being exposed to the open skies. Worse of all though was what this psychologist was going to find out about him and what he might do about it. Section him maybe? Will couldn't rule that out if he banged on too much about Thom.

The tranquillizers were working well. He didn't care about anything too much now. He just had to sit there and let Becks find the place.

But when they'd finally arrived and parked the car things took a turn for the worse.

The surroundings were lovely, just an old-fashioned row of shops in a little village. A butchers', a bakers' and probably a set of candlesticks in the window of the jewellers beside the convenience store.

'You'll be alright darling.' Becks had tried to assure him as she helped him out of the car. But he wasn't alright. He was suddenly struck by that awful feeling of doom again and that fluttering of dread that flowed through the whole of his body. It wasn't making him physically panic as it had before but that was probably because the drugs were doing their bit to ease it.

Still didn't think he could go through with it though, walk up to the heavy black door of the house with its big brass plaque and get summoned in to some grim fate. Meet a perfect stranger and have him attack whatever was left of his mind.

When he admitted this to Becks, his voice trembling, she forcefully told him he had to. He hadn't expected that. He thought she'd be a little more understanding. He'd pretty much expected her to say it was fine and just turn the car around and take him home. But she began crying angry tears and holding the car door open wide.

'Please, Will,' she said, 'you've got to get better.'
It looked like she might collapse. The tears were streaming from her and she was choking on them. Her face screwed into something ugly.

He realized then that for all of the calmness she'd shown before, she was falling apart almost as much as he was. She just wasn't the drama queen he'd turned out to be.

So now he'd do it. He knew he had to, for her and for both of them. All the sorrow she'd risen above to help him had to be reciprocated.

'Sorry sweetheart, I'll go... I'm really sorry... please come here.'
And Will held her for a while, her head bowed beneath his head and his chest.

'Come on then,' she said sniffing her tears away 'or we'll be late.'
He was seriously struggling to walk though. He couldn't feel the tremors in his legs because of the tranquilizers but they were there alright, he could sense them. Still he kept on, step by step, careful and slow and she was right there beside him.

Will still wasn't sure if he was mad or if everyone else was ignorant. If Thom was real what then? He'd let everyone down hadn't he? The whole fucking world. Though in all honesty he thought, fuck everyone else who was going to die, all that mattered for the moment was that Becks would die too and he wanted her to be happy for whatever time was left.

If on the other hand and as he hoped, desperately hoped, Thom had just been a figment of his arsehole mental imagination it was only Becks who'd be left to suffer.

It was clear then that he'd have to do whatever this shrink wanted of him. He'd go with the flow. He'd suffer the cure or suffer all attempts to be cured, if only to bring things to an acceptable conclusion for her.

If he was certifiable there would be a certificate and everyone including himself would have to accept it. Her mum and dad and her friends would all be there for her and eventually the idea would become acceptable to her? He'd try and make it easier for her and then perhaps she could move on?

Eventually she'd have someone normal by her side. She'd have a life and though it killed him to think it, he'd be a distant memory of hers one day.

Becky pressed the bell which rang audibly on the outside and no doubt reverberated throughout the whole of the inside of the building.

Will hung onto the outside wall, the wait seeming endless but eventually the door was opened.

A very tall man with wiry auburn hair stood before them sporting an unkempt beard that was turning to grey. To finish the effect, he was wearing John Lennon glasses. Just the sort of look Becky had expected to see when they visited the psychiatrist.

'Hello,' She said sheepishly. 'We've come for an appointment with Frank O'Keefe.'

'Well you've found him!' He answered in a rich Irish brogue.

'You're William then?' He said to Will with a toothy grin. 'And this'll be your wife? Come in, come in!'

Becky ushered Will in first and followed close behind just in case his awkward shuffling turned into a stagger.

The psychologist reached a door at the end of the hall and opened it.

'Go easy my friend.' He said watching Will struggling to catch him up and when he'd finally passed him into the room he looked at Becky attentively.

'If you don't mind you can go into the waiting room there.' He said pointing to another door.

'There's a toilet if you feel the need and there are the usual magazines you find in waiting rooms on the table. Feel free to use the coffee machine but be warned, rather you than me.'

'Oh and listen... he'll be fine with me my dear.' He said in almost a whisper.

Will was waiting for him just inside his office desperately struggling to stand upright as his anxiety grew.

'Please, sit down my friend.' The psychologist said to Will as he quietly closed the door.

Becks wouldn't have been at all surprised by the décor Will decided. There were just two chairs, both facing each other. Leather armchairs that you could sink into and each had a little wooden table beside them, one with a box of tissues upon it, so Will was at least sure of where he was supposed to sit. There was a kettle on a trolley in the corner with all sorts of condiments beside it. Other than that, there were just a handful of shelves high above them on one side of the room with folders set down haphazardly.

Will finally sunk into his chair while the psychologist waited patiently in his own.

They sat facing each other for some time in silence, Frank's well-meaning glare somewhat disturbing to the patient. Will tried to match him but found himself focusing just below the eyes and above the frames of the glasses.

How much more of this? He wondered but then the Irishman presented him with a charismatic smile.

'Well this is bollocks though isn't it William just sitting here like this?'

Will smiled back in agreement.

'So why is it you're here then?'

'Erm... Doctor Baker thinks it might do me good.' Will answered timidly.

'And what do you think?'

'I've just got to do it haven't I?'

'But do you think you need my help?'

'I'll give it a try.'

'But you're not convinced?'

'I don't know.'

'Okay, that's honest enough.'

The psychologist began to stare again in silence.

Will scratched at his scalp with discomfort.

'You weren't moving terribly well when you came in were you?' Frank suddenly mentioned.

'No, I wasn't.'

'So, do you think it's more of a physical thing or a mental thing with the walking?'

Will fixed on Frank's eyes now as he began feeling a little perturbed.

'What do you think?' He growled.

'Not my legs William.'

More silence.

'Let me just explain then.' Frank said finally. 'It can't be physical because I'm sure there are times when you're perfectly fine and you can move freely. Am I right?'

'Yes.'

'So, it must be something to do with your mind?'

'Yeah I guess.' Will answered disconcertedly.

'Okay, it's good that we're agreed and now you see we have to find out what's wrong inside your head. It won't be anything insurmountable even if you're thinking you're screwed. Trust me you're not.'

Will nodded appreciatively.

Further silence.

Will wondered if he'd been given a cue to start talking as if the ice was meant to have been broken.

'You can call me Will.' He said for want of something to say.

'Thank you Will I shall and I hope you'll just call me Frank.'

'Deal.' Will agreed making the psychologist smile.

'So, Will, Doctor Baker and as I like to call him, Julian, filled me in a little bit about your childhood. It seems to me you had an awful lot to overcome. Losing your brother like that? Just terrible and then your dad going off. But you coped with it alright didn't you? You and your mam?'

Will raised his eyebrows to display his agreement.

But did yer though Will? Really? You see children are incredibly resilient, aren't they? They have this amazing ability to pick themselves up and dust themselves down and just get on with it. Don't you think? Whether it's literally falling over and scraping their knees or watching their daddy wave them goodbye from a car he's never going to come back in. They don't seem to care in any deep sense of the word and just take their new situation for what it is and somehow muddle through. If you let them that is. So, was it like that with you Will?'

'Well I suppose it was.' Will responded having taken a few moments to ponder.

'Like you said, you're really choked for a while but then you just get used to it… you know what I mean? You just adapt.'

'So, there you are Will.' Frank said dismally. 'You're quite a textbook case if I could ever allow myself to think there was such a thing.'

'But what about these visions I've been having?'

'Ah yes.' Frank muttered as he looked down at his notes.

'I think your anxiety has tried to find a channel to escape out from.'

'But they really seem real Frank, I mean really real, like they're *really* happening.'

The psychologist seemed taken aback by Will's sudden veracity. 'Well,' Frank said, 'the mind has a nasty way of playing tricks on you sometimes. It isn't terribly unusual for someone such as yourself to have an over irrational fear of the calamities that might befall us all. Natural disasters, man-made disasters. Fixating on those fears are just your mind's way of deferring the real issues you should be facing. Although I must say it's a bit unusual to have conjured up something quite so intricate. You must have a very vivid imagination.'

'So, you don't think I'm mad?' Will asked, a little more desperately than he'd hoped to sound.

The Psychologist gave a wry smile.

'No, you're not mad my friend... you're just ill.'

Will's eyes began to swell but he was able to check himself in time although the relief on his face was discernible.

'Glad to see a little emotion escaping there Will.' Frank said, studying his patient with soft benevolent eyes and when there was nothing else from him he continued his questions.

'Were you very close to your mam?'

'Yeah, I guess so.'

'And she was affectionate to yer?'

Will threw him a quizzical look.

'What do you mean?' He asked

'Did she hug yer? Give you a cuddle when you were feeling low?'

'Not really... I'm a grown man.' He said with mild irritation.

'When you were a child for heaven's sake?'

'Not much... she wasn't a touchy feely sort of person... she was a great mum though.'

'Okay,' Frank sighed, 'you obviously must of felt a great deal of her to spark how you've been malfunctioning of late.'

'So, my *grieving* has been sending me mad?'

'No not that, I doubt you've been doing a lot of grieving in the expected manner have you? Hardly any I might wager? Which is an awful big part of the reason why you're here now.'

'I don't understand' Will confessed.

Frank produced an empty sheet from the back of his clipboard and began to draw. It was a crude picture of a pint glass. He flipped it up vertically for Will.

'Everyone', he began, 'suffers a certain amount of stress in their life; bad luck, even tragedy. Normally there are ways either consciously or subconsciously to dispel it. You have your family to console you. You have hobbies or even work if you enjoy it. It helps you stay in control. Now look at this.' He said as he scrawled a line a few inches from the bottom of the glass he'd drawn.

'Now that's what you'd expect of a man of your age with any sort of childhood that we'd like to term, just for the sake of argument, normal. That would be the level of stress we'd expect. As you can see it's a long way from the top of the glass.

Now in your case Will... and with so many others like you, the line is so much higher.'

Will watched Frank slash a second line just below the roof of the glass.

'Children have no idea how to handle the stress of life you see? If they're not given help it stays there, boiling toward the surface... and the thing is Will, that they're too close to the edge and if they're not given the help they need when they're young, by the time they're older the strain of everyday life will hit them when they're adults just by experiencing the usual sort of difficulties other adults do.'

Frank paused for dramatic effect.

'Eventually your life spirals out of control and the glass overflows.'

To accompany the explanation Frank drew a line an inch above the glass and the excess falling down with sudden jerks of his pen, all over the wilderness below.

'That's where you are Will. You've fallen over the edge.'

James heard the milk float slowly passing by his window. Never stopped at his building or the ones next door, strange with so many inhabitants? James couldn't help but wonder if the poor milkman had been diddled a few times? *'My husband will pay you next time,'* or *'Our benefit cheque hasn't arrived,'* or more likely with this crowd, *'It was my cousin's responsibility to pay you and she has left to who knows where?'*

A quick flick of the curtains showed it wasn't quite daylight but it was certainly heading towards it and to think he was still drunk by a fairly sizable degree.

Definitely for the best though. Wouldn't want to be sober ever again if he had the choice.

Now what about the face and the ear? Hadn't attempted to look at them for a while and still wasn't sure if the blurred vision was down to the booze or the clout around the head... hilarious!

Still quite blurred but from the reflection it would seem he escaped without so much as a scratch.

The ear certainly had a sting to it if you rubbed it but then the answer would be not to rub it... courtesy of Tommy Cooper... was that one of his?

The lady certainly had a good swing though didn't she? Bang! And James had seen it coming all of the way as if in slow motion, yet his own senses were completely shot by then and he was neither prepared nor capable of dodging the blooming hand so it had landed full on sending him crashing against the wall and all of the way down to the floor.

Didn't even know Brian was present until he'd grabbed him from under an elbow and yanked him up.

It was so incredibly kind of Brian to stand between him and his assailants like that. Every one of them towering above him, the men anyway.

He must have rushed from his room when he heard the commotion.

James just might have let out a bit of a shriek when the lady had taken him down, bloody rings clattering his ear like that... extremely painful.

Then suddenly there were all of these men and youths appearing out of nowhere. By the time Brian had helped him to his feet there must have been at least half a dozen of them and the stupid woman who had actually struck him, was in a complete paddy in the opposing corner, screaming and bawling as if she'd been the one attacked and that strange little old lady, who he had recognised, being that she was wearing the same long *hijab* as always, was hugging her, holding her face between the palms of her hands, chanting... I mean she might really have been chanting by the sounds she was making... absolutely ludicrous.

Where on earth did all of these people come from? How many of them could they squeeze into those small rooms? Where did they all *sleep?* Wasn't allowed surely?

No doubt the landlord would have more than a few things to say about it all if he knew. Not that James would, in the cold light of day, have anything malicious to say against these people.

They had all no doubt escaped some terrible conflict in their homeland and it was an awful comment he'd made about the communal parts of the building being a warzone. Thought he was being clever in his drunken state but perhaps he ought to try being a good deal more charitable next time?

Oh yes! He remembered now, those poor tiny tots... perhaps that demented lady's children? Hadn't really taken much notice of them any time previously as they'd always been swept in and out of the front door or along the path, all in baby buggies and top heavy with shopping bags, but they had been there throughout.

They were literally screaming the place down from the off. One tiny little girl who could barely have been more than two years of age had been jumping up and down, flapping her little hands and just the most extraordinary noise from her poor little lungs.

It didn't seem as if any of the other women who had begun appearing had even given those unfortunate children even a moment's thought, far too busy adding their own voices to that crescendo of sound.

Deborah had introduced and trained him very well in the art of the 'domestic' but what he had been subjected to last night was beyond ridiculous.

Although in retrospect it was Deborah who was inadvertently responsible for starting the whole cycle of events with her hateful, unforgivable revelation.

The revelation that had left him shell shocked, desolate and completely fucking *destroyed.*

Shaking with a crazed paroxysm he was.

Pissed and very conspicuous with it too, it being a Monday, he had sat in the bar and drank pint after pint with enormous urgency in a frantic effort to try and calm down but became more bewildered than calm it would seem.

At one point he tried very briefly to cheer himself up with something other than alcohol by playing a couple of songs on the juke box machine.

First time he'd chosen a tune on one since the days when there were real vinyl records inside dropping onto a turntable... it was all digital now.

Wanted to play something upbeat, take him out of himself for a little while.

Don Mclean's 'American Pie' was an easy choice... always seemed to raise the spirits regardless of the tragic background of the song.

Then he had a second song to choose for the pound investment he'd made.

There was such an enormous choice. James went through what seemed an endless catalogue of music, clinging to the side of the machine and pressing the arrow which made the song choices rotate.

And there he was enjoying the nostalgia that some of the song titles were giving him until he'd seen a face on an album cover that had fed him such striking emotions with its memory.

The man who had sung their wedding song.

Debbie's choice but his as well. It really did feel like their song at the time and how remarkable now to think it ever did.

The record was by the black chap with the dreadlocks, it wasn't Bob Marley but rather the chap who somehow always reminded James of Rod Stewart. He could never remember his name before yesterday and he'd already forgotten it again. Couldn't even remember the title of the song either, not a chance to be honest, but there were a few words that would occasionally resonate.

'All alone with you makes the butterflies in me arise.'
How on earth did he ever feel those sentiments for Deborah? How misguided his loins had made him! Couldn't even begin to comprehend how he had managed to feel so very much for her and now all he was left with was a burning hatred of the woman.

She may well be the mother of his children but he despised her with the sort of misgiving he would never have thought himself capable of.

Lots more to drink then as he sat milling over the absurdity of the marriage and his thoughts on Deborah's final twist of the knife.

How on earth had she even approached it?
How then could you explain to a boy of ten that his father was a sexual pervert?

Would he even have known what one was?
What basic phrases could she have used? Bet she hadn't bothered to get some advice on the subject, well couldn't have could she? Even the most ardent social worker would have her work cut out trying to find anything James had done that could damage a child.

It remained abundantly clear to James that the only damage done was by telling poor Adam those things and for what possible benefit to their son?

Some fuzzy excuse about being stressed by having to defend her reasoning to the boy for blocking the visits! She'd just snapped apparently, but James knew it was pure vindictiveness and that poor little boy who now shunned him was going to suffer terribly for it one way or another.

Oh, but James didn't want to dwell on it just now and fortunately recollecting last night allowed him a little time out of mind.

He rubbed his withered grey hands together to produce some sort of sensation and sighed heavily.

Go on then, let's invoke some more of the details of last night he instructed the forlorn figure in his reflection.

He vaguely remembered being asked to leave the pub yet couldn't quite recall why and then he'd stumbled his way into the convenience store and bought some of the strong cider that came in cans. Not much more than that until the incident.

As far as he was aware he had just returned to the room to continue drinking himself into a stupor. Had no recollection of trying to talk his way through Brian's door and surely even in his most smashed condition he'd be wary of trying something like that after the short shrift he'd been given of late and rightly so.

The real shame was last night's escapade had almost certainly put paid to any sort of relationship he and Brian had left.

Still couldn't place the time he had appeared like a Knight in tartan armour?

So, the woman and the man were in the hall literally howling at each other, toddlers screaming the place down and then came the slamming of the front door. Irritating when it was an accident, especially as much of the time it was sheer thoughtlessness, but the door was slammed again and again. It would seem the man was attempting to leave, the woman pulling him back, a minute's respite then, slam! All over again!

Wouldn't have got involved under any normal circumstance however upsetting or alarming he found it... not very courageous when it came to confrontation, but of course he'd been drinking an inordinate amount of very strong cider.

Even then he had done his utmost to ignore it but then one last slam and that infernal woman shrieking like that and he just found himself bounding out of his door all guns blazing and giving her a piece of his mind.

It was just he and she for the moment save the little ones, but then the front door swung back open and the husband, partner or whoever had rushed back in and yes! that was it... James had glanced behind him for just a split second and when he turned back he saw the stupid woman's hand flying through the air at him and out of the corner of his eye Brian standing there in his doorway.

So *that* was when he'd arrived.

Bless him for helping him to his feet like that and fending off all of them so bravely, calling for calm and even pushing one or two of them back very gently with a hand.

If only it could have stopped there.

'Come on let's get some air.' Brian had suggested to ease the situation and he'd helped James stagger onto the front step and James was sure, really quite certain that Brian had slipped and fallen of his own accord.

He had kept trying to ascertain the facts over and over in the hospital, but Brian wasn't at all interested in talking to him then. Didn't actually want James to stay with him but how in blazes could he not?

He could see Brian was in an awful lot of pain but at least it wasn't a break or even a fracture, just a sprain.

The nurse said he'd be limping around for a week or two but then she was sure he'd make a full recovery.

James had been so relieved.

Had to wonder though, as he looked his reflection square in the face... how on earth was *he* ever going to recover after yesterday?

If truth be told he didn't think he could.

Will could walk unaided now, albeit shakily. The drugs prescribed clearly doing their job.

Made him wonder all the more why he was back outside Frank's door.

The trouble is he'd been a complete sycophant when Doctor Baker had asked how the first meeting had gone.

'Was it useful?' The doctor had asked.

'I think so.' Will had lied.

'So, you're happy to visit him again?'

'Definitely.' Will had said and he had been so pleased he was sitting next to Becks when he'd said it just so that they couldn't make eye contact, because his answer was quite a bit more enthusiastic than what he'd implied to her it might be. He'd actually told her he couldn't really see the point of it all but at least he conceded that he would carry on if she wanted him too.

Why he'd told Doctor Baker something so completely different he couldn't tell. Perhaps it was his accent or maybe he didn't want to disappoint him being how kind and knowledgeable he was.

It didn't matter now. He was outside the fucking place and when he'd finished smoking he was going to have to ring on the bell if Becks didn't beat him to it.

'How are yer Will? Frank asked once he'd led him to his office, giving him one of his big smiles.

'Well, you know... alright.' Will said without much conviction.

'Ah Good.' Frank said. 'But your knees are shaking some Will.'

'Yes, I know.'

'That says to me you're suffering.'

'You're right, I am a bit.' Will admitted.

'It isn't nice to see.' Frank observed.

'I'm sorry.'

'God! Don't be sorry... I'm just telling you that sitting here watching someone in distress like you are is upsetting for me.'

'I'm improving though,' Will pointed out, 'the drugs are beginning to kick in.'

'Yes, the drugs,' Frank said, 'but where do you think you'll be if you stop taking them?'

'Not sure.'

'Ah, but I am Will. You're already with the shakes there and if you take away the medication you'll be terribly anxious again.'

'You were a wreck Will.'

'Okay.'

'That is why you need to persist with these sessions my friend. You'll find it'll work if you make the effort.'

'Fire away then.' Will said nonchalantly.

'You know I'm going to ask you about your brother don't you?'

'Thought you might.'

'So, tell me then Will, what was his name?'

'Matthew, though we always called him Matt.'

'Ah right, so you were always Will?'

'No. Everyone called me Billy when I was a boy.'

'I see, so you changed it to something a bit more sophisticated when you got older?'

'Something like that yeah.'

Frank smiled his indulgence.

'And did you get on, the pair of you?'

'Yeah, really well,' Will enthused, 'he was my big brother, I idolized him.'

'Right, of course… good. So, what was the age gap then?'

'Well, I was eight and he had just turned eleven.'

'Must have been terribly painful for you when he went?'

Will simply shrugged his shoulders.

'So, tell then Will, what was the cause of your brothers' death?'

'He was run over.' Will said sedately.

'Ah shit that's awful!' Frank moaned. 'On the way to school? On the way home?'

'No, we were playing out.'

'Fuck! So you were *with* him?'

'Yeah.' Will confirmed.

He was beginning to feel uncomfortable and he clasped the palms of his hands together against his lips as he began to feel a little breathless.

'Tell me about it.' Frank asked.

'Really?' Will sighed.

'Yes please.'

Will took a deep breath. He could feel the ache in the pit of his stomach begin like he always did whenever he began to think properly about Matt. He moved his hands down onto his jeans and rubbed them gently up and down as he tried to find the words to begin.

Frank eyed him patiently.

When Will finally tried to speak he was surprised to find how he was spluttering his words incomprehensively.

'Just take your time.' Frank advised softly.

'Sorry.' Will gasped as he struggled for composure.

'The last thing you need to be is sorry.' Frank assured him. 'Go on, keep trying... I know it must be difficult.'

Will cleared his throat and shook his head.

'I'm not normally like this.' He said disconcertedly.

'Just go on.' Frank said looking at his patient sternly.

Minutes passed, long agonising minutes before Will made a start.

'We were playing a game,' he began finally, 'just me and Matt... Matt was always making up these silly games...' he continued, with just a flicker of a smile, 'he always used to beat me at them as well... what with being that much older and always changing the rules as he went along.'

Frank caught Will's eye and they grinned an allegiance.

'So anyway, we were playing this game,' he explained again, 'just the pair of us, it was the middle of the Summer holidays and we were bored shitless. It was so hot that day and we'd just been sitting around in the garden annoying each other, fighting each other for the swing, arguing about everything and nothing and generally driving my mum to distraction... anyway, she got sick of having to leave the housework every five minutes to stop the pair of us attacking each other. *'It's a lovely day,'* she said *'go to the park or somewhere'*, basically she was telling us to sling our hooks and get out from under her feet, so we did.

Course we couldn't be bothered to go to the park as it really was a scorcher of a day and it wasn't the sort of park you could kick a ball about in so we just went to the end of the road where the A1 runs down to the city right under the Archway Bridge if you know it?'

'I don't I'm afraid.' Frank answered.

'Oh,' Will said with surprise, 'an Irishman that doesn't know North London! Oh well,' he sighed, 'it's quite a famous bridge in North London; amazing views of the city up there but its best known for the jumpers.'

'God suicides!' Frank gasped.

'Yeah.' Will confirmed solemnly. 'So much so, no one calls it Archway Bridge, it's always been Suicide Bridge for as long as I've known it.'

'And what about the poor buggers driving along below?' Frank asked.

'I know... I've often wondered about them myself... although the guy who got Matt wasn't... er...'

Will's speech suddenly wavered and although he was shaping his lips in the shape of the words his tongue had ceased to move and he darted his eyes quickly away from Frank's view as unbecoming tears welled up in his eyes.

'Shit! So, Matt died there on that road.' Frank said gravely.
Will sniffed hard and blinked away the tears but continued to stare vacantly at the wall.

Frank sat back calmly and watched intently as Will gradually managed to suppress the worst of his emotions.

'It's good.' Frank informed him solemnly, yet Will felt both ashamed and ridiculous.

'Fucksake!' Will moaned, eventually managing to reprimand himself.

'But you *need* to grieve Will.' Frank said. 'Billy should have done a whole lot of crying and if you can't cry for yourself then at least shed some tears for little Billy.'

Will nodded in obedience and let the silent tears roll down his face.

'Good man,' Frank whispered, 'and whenever you're ready you can tell me the rest.'

Chapter 34 – Matt's death

The boys sat side by side on the concrete wall as the traffic streamed down the slope from under the bridge bringing with it the dust and grit and a welcomed breeze.

They had decided to play the letter game that Matt had made up in the weeks before.

Both would choose a letter that would appear on the end of a car registration and the first to count a hundred of their chosen letter on the cars that passed downhill won the game.

'I'm gonna be M.' Billy said.

'I knew you'd say that.' Matt replied scornfully.

'It's fair though Matt.' Billy countered.

'I know, but it doesn't mean to say you'll definitely win.'

'So! I know it doesn't,' Billy agreed, 'but it's more fairer.'

'I don't see why we can't have more letters though.' Matt argued.

'Cos I don't want to; we can have more letters in the next game.'

'Alright.' Matt agreed grudgingly. 'But don't stop playing if your losing this time.'

'I won't.' Billy said, confident he'd win.

'I'm gonna be L's then.'

'Okay.'

'Shall we start now then?' Matt asked quickly.

Billy squinted his eyes at the cars coming down the hill in the distance.

'No!' he said firmly.

'You're just saying that 'cos there's an L coming!' Matt said angrily.

'I know I am... why don't we start in one minute's time like normal?' Billy suggested.

'Fine!' Matt agreed holding his wrist up to show Billy his watch. 'Let the big hand get to twelve then we'll start a minute after that.'

Both boys studied the hand of the watch intently as it made a circuit around the face.

There was a wall of cars beneath them as the game began.

'One!... two!' Billy counted as they watched the cars descend around the curve in the road that led down to a junction with traffic lights.

'One!' Matt countered as the next wave of vehicles passed.

'Three!... four!' Billy responded.

'Where's four?'

'Look, that yellow Cortina.' Billy said pointing it out and Matt resentfully agreed.

Billy was already winning the game by a score of four to one, a lead he was never destined to lose even though the confirmation of points scored from his brother came ever more grudgingly and open to debate.

'Sixty-seven against fifty-two.' Billy said cheerfully on the last count.

'I know!' Matt snarled. 'You don't have to keep saying it!'

There was a lull in the traffic at the time. The gaps in the road periodic due to the lights further up the hill toward Highgate. Then there would be a sudden surge; columns of vehicles converging into two lanes, racing each other to the next set of lights.

'Fifty-three, fifty-four, fifty-five!' Matt shouted triumphantly as the cars passed below.

'Sixty-eight, sixty-nine!' Billy responded above the noise.

'No way!' Matt screamed his disagreement.

'Yes it is! That gold Capri and that big white car!'

'That white one was an N!' Matt protested.

'It was an M cheater!'

'No!' Matt screamed again having the last word.

It was the last word Billy or anyone else would ever hear his brother speak.

In a fraction of a second Matt had leapt the six feet or so from the wall to race toward the central reservation where he might get a better view of the white car which was trapped for the moment in a bottle neck of vehicles as the cars swung left at the lights.

He'd barely noticed the Volvo trailing so far behind the rest of the traffic.

He hadn't noticed it switch lanes to the one that ran beside the thin stretch of curb he'd just leapt down to, falling forward as he did into the road from the momentum of landing.

Billy watched him fly across the bonnet and against the wall. He saw the car skid sideways to a halt. He looked down at his brother motionless in the road, arms splayed, legs twisted, eyes fixed blankly at the sky.

Billy calmly turned and hung carefully from the wall then let himself drop.

He stood waiting for the man who'd just got out of the car who was walking a bit wobbly.

Billy was frightened. He knew they were going to get really told off and he was going to have to say sorry for him and his brother.

Panic gripped him and he ran and he ran.

The whole apartment awash with sunlight almost as hazy as he was.
Becks had to go to work after a while.
He accepted it, course he did. Made her sad though, but he kept
telling her he was fine.
Her mum popped in a lot. 'Just popping in.' She'd say bless her.
She was always fussing about his food but he didn't want to eat
most of the time.
Made him even more tired than normal, eating did.
'You're supposed to before you take your pills.' She'd remind him.
Thom had gone and mum was there, dad too sometimes; once
all four of them, the whole family walking around the duck pond in
Waterlow Park.
He was chasing Matt as he kicked the ball that rustled and spread
the damp brown leaves under the trees.
The leaves outside the apartment are bright green mostly,
caught by the sun.
The green Van Gogh would try to capture whenever he painted
trees.
It could be roasting in the lounge but he just soaked it up, too
tired to move.
Becks brought him in cigarettes anyway.
'I'm always catching you watching Pingu.' Her mum said
laughing.
Didn't even know it was on.
He liked to listen to the radio mainly.
It was nice to get up with Becks and listen to Radio One while she
dashed about getting ready for work.
Must have felt like a quick day for her when she was chasing
about like that, but it was such a long one for him, until she came
home.

Chapter 36 - The things that people do in the dark

James felt he had no other choice but to besiege Brian's room if he were to have a chance to speak with him one last time.

He'd already knocked on his door twice earlier in the day which he was sure was a decent enough hour for Brian to be up or at least awake... it certainly was the second time, but Brian had obviously chosen not to answer.

James couldn't blame him for that, not after all of his antics and he didn't want the poor man to think he was stalking him, but James really wanted to explain things before he left.

He needed to leave Brian with at least a half decent impression of the man he had once been and to offer some sort of explanation as to why he'd become the drunken wreck that Brian was far more familiar with.

James was sober now of course. Clean and smart too for a change.

He was hoping *last* impressions would also count for something.

When Brian did finally emerge, James was ready for him. He had simply been sitting at the end of his bed with the door ajar just enough to see his friend shuffling out of his own door.

He quickly rested the book he'd been reading and dashed out into the hall to nab him.

It was awful to see Brian physically wince at the sound of his own name and when he had turned around he noted the seriousness of his pallor, clearly steeling himself for an unpleasant confrontation.

'I only want to keep you for a minute!' James had said hurriedly. 'You see I'm leaving today which is why I've been waiting for you... I was rather hoping I could have a few final words before I set off?'

Brian's stern expression quickly lightened to that of surprise and James was able to usher him into his room while his friend's mind was still processing the unexpected news.

'Look.' He said eagerly, as he pointed at the zipped-up suitcase lying flat in the middle of the bed.

'Oh.' Brian gasped.

'Yes, you see I really am leaving.'

'So where are ye off to then?'

'Well...' James hesitated, I'm not quite sure yet ... something similar I should imagine just somewhere else... give you a bit of peace!'

'Come on!' Brian exclaimed. 'You don't want to be leaving on account of me!'

'No old chap,' James was quick to counter, 'nothing to do with you if I'm being perfectly honest. I just thought a change would do me good.'

'Aye,' Brian reasoned after a moment, 'perhaps yer wise.'

'I think so.' James concluded.

'Anyway, the reason I called you in was obviously to say goodbye but I'd also like to explain my recent behaviour and hopefully explain the rather spineless stance I've taken with my wife.'

'No, no, no... listen,' Brian had remonstrated as James attempted his opening speech, 'ye don't have to explain a thing to me old pal.'

'But please I'd like to!' James asserted.

'If not for your sake then at least for mine. You see I'd like to give my side of the story and to be perfectly honest I can't think of anyone else to give it to.'

'Can I just close this first?' He asked as he slid past Brian and pushed the door to.

'It's all to do with sex you see.' He said nonchalantly.

'Now James...' Brian said holding up his hand as a barrier in an attempt to curtail any further revelation.

'Please,' James said sternly, 'you've had me screaming the place down and crying on your doorstep so I don't see how my laying myself bare like this could be any worse. We are both men after all and men are known to discuss the sexual side of nature.'

Brian lowered his hand and nodded in his reluctance.

'You see, I've had trouble getting it up.' James began in earnest. 'Have done for years. I know there's a multitude of drugs you can take for it now but I've always suffered with low blood pressure so I've been advised that it's best not to.'

Brian listened in bemusement.

'You see Deborah, my wife, has always been rather keen on the whole sex thing. An amazing libido for a woman and if truth be told

I could never keep up with her, even in my younger days and as time went on and my ability to perform decreased she became more and more frustrated. She was sympathetic at first and we tried all sorts of holistic things to remedy the situation but eventually she lost all compassion.'

'I think her yearning for sex being as great as it was she began to perceive me as a hopeless case and bought herself one of those contraptions that left me pretty much superfluous... then we began sort of drifting apart; quite rapidly in fact. Bickering about everything and anything. You see I had frustrations of my own.'

James chose to pause there for a moment having noticed how uncomfortable Brian had become.

'I'm so sorry,' he said, 'I'm coming to the point I promise you... anyway yes... you see it got to the point where whenever we argued my masculinity would be called into question. Even if I had a problem installing a new appliance she would happily concur that I wasn't man enough rather than agree there was a more rational explanation.'

Brian remained silent. His eyes now firmly fixed on the suitcase and away from James' scrutiny.

'Well, it all came to a head,' James continued, 'when I quite foolishly put an ad in one of those contact magazines.'

'Totally without Deborah's knowledge you understand.' He added in an instant as Brian's bewildered eyes flicked upward for a moment.

'I was so bloody desperate by then you see. For the both of us really, because although I couldn't... still can't in fact, manage much myself, a man still has his needs. Do you understand that Brian?'

'Aye.'

'Well, as I said, I was stupid enough to place an add asking to meet other couples in our area. I'd naturally put that I myself would be a non-participant although if things progressed as I hoped they would I was expecting that to change you see?'

Brian, James observed, looked almost queasy now or decidedly ill at ease in any case.

'I can see I've shocked you,' he continued undeterred, 'although not half as much as it shocked my wife so it transpires. She absolutely hit the roof. My suitcase was packed and I was out of the door that very same evening.'

'I still can't decide if she was truly offended or if it was simply the excuse she needed to finally be rid of me. Either way, here I am and have been since... until today of course.'

'You may have surmised that the nature of my leaving left me in the situation where I lost what small amount of friends I had, or rather we had, not to mention my entire family disowning me. Deborah had been very quick to broadcast my wrong-doing to all and sundry but at least she had kept it from the children as I'd expect any decent mother should.'

'Until the day of that episode of ours?' Brian finally piped up. 'Yes' James replied, suddenly struggling for composure.

'Aye, well I'm very sorry for yer troubles old boy.' Brian said solemnly.

'Oh well, James chirped, trying to sound a little more cheerful, 'what's done is done... I just wanted you to know.'

'Yer needn't have.'

'Well to be honest Brian, It's made me feel a lot better getting it off of my chest and hearing the whole thing out loud rather than just milling it around in my head.'

'And yer not decided where it is yer off to?' Brian enquired. 'Not yet... some sort of B&B to begin with I expect, until I find somewhere more permanent.'

The two men faced each other now, James rocking on his heels and giving his friend an indulgent smile.

'Are you certain you have to go?' Brian asked despondently. 'Oh yes, absolutely certain.'

'Then I'll wish yer all the very best.' Brian said in earnest as he offered James his hand to shake.

'Thank you so much Brian,' James replied, clearly moved and squeezing the hand tightly.

'I want to thank you very much for your friendship and support and I'll always remain mortified about your ankle.'

'Oh come on… it's history.' Brian uttered as he shifted slowly toward the door, gently wriggling from James's grasp.

James shuffled over to let his friend out.

'All the best then.' Brian said again.

'And to you sir.' James countered as he quietly closed the door.

Chapter 37 - The last appointment

'Make yourself comfortable.' Frank said. 'I must say you're looking amazingly better... and how long has it been since you last came to see me? Just over a fortnight is it?'

'Yes.' Will said cheerfully.

'And no Mrs Shepherd today, so I take it you drove yourself here?'

'Yep... legs are working properly again thank god.'

'And no more visits from your friend from the past?'

'No, he's gone now I think.' Will said with a smile. 'Not sure where to... although he did say something about getting carted off to jail.'

'Good to know he's leaving yer in peace.'

'It certainly is.'

'I must say you've made one hell of a speedy recovery, much quicker than myself or Doctor Baker could ever have envisaged.'

'Those wonderful drugs.' Will declared happily.

'Oh, but so much more than that Will, you opening up like you did last time would have done yer a power of good.'

Will grimaced.

'I'm so pleased I won't have to go through that again.' He said meekly.

'It's such an important thing to release those emotions.' Frank asserted.

'I'm sure.' Will said shifting in his chair. 'I'm just pleased I don't have to go through that embarrassment again.'

'Is it that embarrassing to show your emotions then?' Frank asked.

'It's horrible.' Will said.

'I'm not afraid of my emotions Will.' Frank professed proudly.

'Good for you.' Will replied impetuously while absentmindedly reaching into his shirt pocket for his cigarettes.

Frank cleared his throat to get Will's attention and pointed at the no smoking sign on the wall.

'Fuck yes! Sorry.' Will said with a grin as he pulled back his hand and lay it on his lap.

'It's not like you to swear though Will is it?'

'I have my moments.' Will confessed as he stared contemptuously into the psychologist's eyes.

Frank chose to pause there and made a point of being seen to physically relax. Eventually he began to speak again and calmly made an observation.

'I wanted to go back to your childhood again but I seem to be getting on your nerves a bit today Will.'

Will didn't know what to say to that. He watched Frank's eyes bearing down on him.

'It's strange how you were perfectly composed when you came in and the moment I start talking about your emotions you get a bit agitated?'

'So, what can I do?' Will asked with a sigh. 'I've never been one to wallow.'

'That's because you're so bloody tough so you are! And look how far it got you!'

Will fixed Frank a menacing look.

'I'm not going to start feeling sorry for myself now... I thought we'd done all that the previous times?'

'We made a start but there are other things to discuss.'

'I don't want to do it again Frank!'

'Then you won't ever get truly better.' The psychologist said bluntly.

'I already am Frank, you said it yourself.'

'Okay, sure,' Frank agreed, 'the drugs have kicked in and given you some balance but it won't be enough. If you don't try to embrace your feelings the psychosis will come back. I wish I was wrong and I wish I could tell you when, but the fact is if you don't deal with your troubles now those demons will all come back and get you.'

'Right then!' Will said flippantly. 'Let's crack on with the misery!'

'And what a big man you are!' Frank said furiously. 'But then what about that little boy you used to know? Can you not feel anything more for him at all? So, we established little Billy lost his big brother... his hero, right there in front of him on that terrible day...

his poor little body mangled? How must Billy have been feeling then when he knew his hero and his best friend in the world wouldn't be playing anymore games? He must have thought in some peculiar way it was his own fault too? Practically tricked Matt into getting himself killed didn't he think? Did anyone tell him otherwise?'

Will bowed his head and kept his eyes fixed on his shoes.

'So, tell me now what it was like in the weeks and months after Will?'

Will shifted uncomfortably in his chair, reeling slightly from the verbal assault.

'Well?' Frank persisted.

'I don't remember that much.' Will said truthfully. 'I suppose I blocked a lot of it out. Although I remember the next Christmas was awful.'

'And how were you feeling then?'

'Terrible.'

'And how were your parents feeling?'

'My dad was gone.'

'Of course he was, I'd forgotten. Then what about your mam?'

'Well, obviously you know the score.'

'Was she upset?'

'Well of course she was upset.'

'And how did she show it?'

'How do you mean?'

'How did she show that she was upset?'

'I don't know.' Will answered.'

'Did she cry on Christmas Day?'

'No.'

'Was there a turkey dinner?'

'Course.'

'Were there decorations?'

'Yes.'

'Did she mention how much she missed your brother and even your dad?'

'No.'

'Then how do you know she was upset?'

'Of *course* she was!' Will said angrily. 'We were both upset.'

'But she thought it best not to show it?'

'I suppose so.'

'For your sake?'

'Yes!'

'Please don't get angry with me.' Frank pleaded. 'I just want to get a picture of how life was for you after your brother had died.'

'Okay.' Will said solemnly.

'So, things continued pretty much as normal.' Frank offered at length.

'Yes, I suppose they did.'

'And how did that make you feel?'

Will wondered then what all this might be leading to.

'It didn't make me feel anything.' He said.

'Okay,' said Frank, 'so you both did your best to carry on as if nothing had happened?'

'Pretty much.'

'Like nothing *terrible* had happened?'

'We just carried on because there wasn't much choice was there? What the fuck else were we supposed to do?'

'I think you were supposed to grieve.' Frank said plainly, ignoring Will's cursing.

He sat quietly for a minute contemplating his patient who was visibly upset now.

'So, are you finished?' Will asked.

'No.' Frank answered.

'What then?' Will wondered holding up his hands in dismay.

'How long did your father stick around for?'

'Don't remember.' Will said frivolously.

'So roughly, was it months, or a year, or several years?'

'It was just a week or two.'

'Then you do remember.'

'Yes.'

'Okay.' Frank said softly. 'I'm sorry but these little details are important Will.'

Will nodded his compliance and Frank noted how flushed he had become.

'Have you any idea why your father left?' He said gently.

'I didn't at the time.'

'But you do now?'

'Oh come on!' Will moaned impatiently, 'it didn't take me long to come up with the notion that it might have had something to do with Matt being gone.'

'When you were a child?'

'Yes.'

'But it was never spoken about?'

'Not to me.'

'Never?'

'Well mum explained that he had gone and that was about it.'

'Nothing else?'

'No.'

'And would you say you were close to your father?'

'I thought I was.'

'But he or your mother never chose to explain why he was leaving?'

'I was eight years old!'

'But doesn't an eight-year old deserve an explanation?'

'Probably, but you're not taking into account how my parents were feeling at the time!' Will suddenly shouted. 'Dad must have been a complete fucking mess!'

'But did either of them ever explain to you how they were feeling?'

'Well clearly my father didn't as I haven't seen him since!'

'But your mother?'

'No Frank, she didn't.'

'And why not?'

'Because I never asked her!'

'Okay, so you didn't ask her and you were only eight, but then you were nine, then you were ten, fifteen, twenty! And don't you think it might have been her that needed to speak to you first?'

Will stooped low in his chair and began shaking his head furiously.

Frank stopped then. He could see how distressed Will had become and he didn't want to push him any harder.

'Anyway, Frank sighed, adjusting his tone, 'would you say your old mam was there for you?'

'What do you mean?'

'Did she comfort you?'

'Well yeah, I'm sure she did.'

'But you don't remember?'

'Look I was only eight Frank, I barely remember those days.'

'Take a tissue.' Frank suggested.

Will clawed at the box on the table beside him and took a clump of tissues. He padded his eyes then blew his nose.

'The thing that troubles me Will,' Frank said in earnest, 'Is I'd be very surprised if your mam didn't hold you close to her whenever you'd been crying and seek you out to comfort you when you were quiet and when you were alone with your thoughts... but if you don't remember it's because it didn't happen.'

'She did her best.' Will said through muffled tears.

'Oh Jesus Will, what about Billy? It must have been terrible to be eight years old and have no one to comfort you?'

'My mum did comfort me!'

'But you don't remember it?'

Will was incensed by the allegation and he wished then he could get up out of his chair to have a swipe at the Irish bastard but instead a more dignified response came to him.

'She had it far worse than me sport.' He said venomously.

'Oh really?' Frank asked with spontaneity, 'and how was that?'

'Well,' he said faltering, 'she... she had me to look after didn't she... on her own and she suddenly had to pay all the bills!'

'Of course! She paid the bills bless her! She didn't let you down did she? No of course not... she knew exactly what to do to make it all better didn't she? Just ignore it all eh? What a fucking genius plan. Get that broom out and sweep every piece of shit, every piece of her own and her little boy's broken heart straight under the carpet. Just go about your business and get the bills paid. That surely must have worked eh? Billy must have appreciated it. No more sad thoughts, no more dark and lonely nights were there? Wonderful! 'I bet you were given treats weren't yer? Sweets, a bike, cinema tickets? I bet life was just grand! But tell me Will... how did that little boy ever climb out of bed in the morning?'

'You don't know anything! Will screamed.

Frank witnessed his patient visibly crumbling before him and he was even howling now.

'Stop.' Will pleaded between gasps of air, his voice fading to a whisper.

'Fine I will.' Frank agreed benevolently as he looked up at the wall clock behind Will's head and straightened his pen.

After a time Will regained his composure and silently accepted the glass of water the psychologist offered to him and when Frank walked him to the front door of the surgery he shook his hand affectionately before leaving.

'Well how did it go?' Becky asked as he came into the apartment and took off his shoes.

'Alright.' Will answered casually. 'Done it now and I don't have to go back again.'

Chapter 38 – A nice drive to Hampstead

It was nice to have a lie in together on a Saturday morning Becky mused.

The sun was shining through the curtains and she was all warm and snugly wrapped in the duvet and crouched beneath Will's head.

She was horny too.

When he woke up she was going to have an expedition down below to see if everything was still working. See how long a little tickle with her finger would get him standing to attention.

Suddenly the phone rang shattering the peace and startling Will awake.

Within a moment he had picked it up and was mumbling his name thickly into the receiver.

He listened to whoever it was for a while and by his body language seemed to be pleased with whatever this person was saying.

'Yeah that's great.' He said eventually, his throat still bunged up with the night's sludge.

'Don't worry I will.' He said excitedly.

'What time? Good...yes fine... brilliant... thank you!'

Will put down the receiver and beamed.

'What was that about?' Becky asked.

'That was the Aston dealers to say my car's ready to pick up. I have to take in my driving licence and fill in a couple of forms then I can drive it away.'

'Oh god! Their admin people are on the ball aren't they!' Becky said sarcastically.

'The thing is I never cancelled it Becks.'

'For heaven's sake Will you idiot!' She moaned.

I didn't really see the point when I'd already paid the deposit.'

'But you get the deposit back don't you?'

'Course you don't Becks, it's a deposit!' That's the whole point, its non-refundable.'

'Christ! How much was that you've lost then?'

'Don't ask... it was a lot... I mean a fucking lot.'

'But you're going to tell them now that you don't want it?'
'But I do want it.'
'Right Will, stop being an absolute prat and phone them back and tell them you can't afford it and you don't want it!'

Becky was completely upright now and rigid with indignation. Will started to laugh. 'I was only winding you up,' He smirked.

'Oh, ha ha!' She said, flopping back under the covers.

Will took a moment to look through the window and across at the trees that had still managed to hold most of their leaves, still pondering how to pose the question he had been hankering to ask her.

'Go on, what are you thinking?' She asked having recognised his look.

'Just that maybe we should buy the thing and sell it again... might get some of the deposit back?'

'God sake!' She groaned bolting upright again. 'And is this you changing your ways is it?' She sneered holding her head in dismay.

'I'll tell you what then,' he said mischievously, 'it's such a beautiful day out there why don't we just pick it up and take it for a spin for a couple of hours?'

'Look Will, stop being a moron and just phone them up.'

'No listen we really can. The guy who sold it to me said if you're not satisfied with it for whatever reason you can bring it back.'

'Don't suppose it ever happens but you're allowed to.'

'And what do you reckon you're going to say when you take it back?'

'Easy, I'll just say I've had a think about it and it turns out I can't afford it... Come on sweetheart! I'll let you drive it!'

'That'll be nice if I crash it... or you do for that matter!'

'So what? I'm insured and he said I could drive it away.'

Becky got out of bed then, shaking her head despondently but Will came bearing down on her and grabbed her hands as she tried to push him away.

'Come on please! Come on sweetheart! Let's do it! Let's go for a nice long drive!' He pleaded as he bounced excitedly before her.

'You're stupid.'

'Oh come on! Please! Please! *Please!* Come on you beautiful, gorgeous, amazing little bird!' He whooped as he caressed her and swung her around.

'Please let's do it Becks?'

'Let go of me then! Let... go of me and we'll do it.' She puffed.

Will let her go and he was wearing the broadest of grins now.

'You're such a fool,' she said, 'we're gonna get into trouble.'

'We won't, I promise... now go and have your shower.'

****

'Where are we going?' She asked when she came out of the bathroom with her hair wrapped in a towel.

'If you don't mind I want to take you for a spin up to Hampstead. It'll be beautiful up there today... Frank wanted me to go as well. Didn't I tell you?'

'Why Hampstead?'

'Well it's just the old stomping ground really... you know, Hampstead Heath, Highgate... where me and Matt used to play. Said it might do some good to see our old house too and you know... see where he died.'

Becky looked at him with rueful eyes.

'I don't know what use it is really but I said I'd do it.'

'Closure.' Becky said solemnly.

'I guess.' Will agreed. 'Good word.'

'Why today though?' Becky asked, 'with the car? Won't there be a lot of traffic?'

'Probably.'

'Then why?'

'I don't know... actually I do know... I really don't wanna go Becks... but it might be easier in a smart convertible mightn't it?'

'And I'll be with you.' Becky said tenderly.

'I know you will darling and that's why I love you so much.'

'What shall I wear?' She asked.

'Ooh I don't know. It's a lovely day but even so the wind'll blow us all over the shop when the hood's down; summer dress and cardi?'

'No, you're right I'll be cold... jeans and Barbour me thinks.'

'And I'll dress like James Bond.'

They took a cab up to the showroom in Brentwood. Will cradling Becky's little fists in his hands and pressing them tightly to his stomach to quell his excitement.

It took a good deal longer than expected to deal with the paperwork.

Becky sat in the guest partition sipping the complimentary coffee and fretting about exactly what it was Will was signing, but when he called her and she saw the car her fears were instantly forgotten.

'It's beautiful.' She gushed as she sat on the leather seating and stroked it gently to feel its softness.

'I love the colour of these seats.'

'Truffle cream.' He said proudly.

'And what's the car?'

'Mercury Silver.'

'It's so beautiful.' She purred as he started the engine and swept the car off of the forecourt onto the road and down the hill toward the M25.

Chapter 39 – A journey to the past

James got on the train at Seven Kings. It was such a glorious day weather wise. Perhaps even the last hurrah of summer?

It suited him very well to remain in the same season. A change in the climate might bring with it a change of heart, but as it was his resolve had stayed intact.

He'd dropped off the suitcase in the Macmillan shop which they'd accepted gratefully. He was grateful himself and might even say it had been a weight off his mind to have the weight quite literally off of his hands. By the time he'd lumbered the case all of that way from the rooms to the High Street he was absolutely exhausted and once he'd reached the station he was looking forward to a good sit down.

The carriage was unexpectedly busy considering it was a Saturday, at least as far as his expectations were concerned. No commuters and he was pretty sure the West Ham boys were playing at a different team's ground but even so he had to sit on the side of the carriage where the low sun kept catching his eyes.

Fortunately, it was a lot more civilised once he arrived at Liverpool Street which he surmised would not be the case on a weekday morning. But thankfully today there wasn't anyone biting at the bit to jump out of the carriage and dash off down the platform to the heady position they enjoyed in whatever financial institution it was they worked in.

However, the next part of the journey felt terribly depressing and in many ways drew a parallel with his own recent existence.

The walk from Liverpool Street Station across just a little piece of the square mile and along the London Wall which was usually so full of movement and life, now, on the weekend, stood empty and well... desolate. The cafés closed, the office space vacated, the sense of abandonment almost palpable.

It was quite a relief to escape that awful atmosphere even if it meant entering the sticky heat of Moorgate Underground Station and waiting then on the platform until the slow rush of dusty warm air brought a tube train.

The Northern line orifice such a very tight fit for the trains that passed through it and there again perhaps his life's recurring problem? He couldn't help but regard everything in a sexual context.

The carriage was so crowded and stiflingly hot it was almost unbearable, yet of course you bore it as did the many thousands of commuters forced to do so each day. Some of them all the way from Barnet and down through Finchley. Not that far for him though thankfully. Eight stops to Hampstead on the Edgware train.

It was still much too early to arrive at Highgate and why the rush being as committed as he was?

Anyway, it was already planned. He'd stop at Hampstead first, indulge one last happy memory; A slow walk up the hill and past all of the lovely old pubs. Definitely wouldn't be stopping off at any of them, although if ever a drop of Dutch courage was required it was very much today.

Nevertheless, the last thing he wanted to happen was for the coroner's report to say he was inebriated.

Will headed northbound and opened up the engine. They were both blown away by the imposing noises it made each time he pressed on the accelerator. The sudden surge of wind swept back their hair and smoothed their faces.

'What do you think?' He shouted over to Becky.

'It's brilliant! It's a monster isn't it?'

Will clung to the thick leather wheel and switched lanes, threading his way through the traffic and grinning dementedly as he passed all before him.

'It's really smooth as well!' Becky screeched in excitement.

'Scary!' Will shouted back. 'It's got so much power it's hard to handle when you're not used to it!'

'He couldn't be that scared Becky thought seeing how he still had that lunatic grin on his face.

Soon they were at the junction that joined them with the M11. It meant less traffic and a much straighter road.

'How nice is this!' Will enthused and Becky could feel herself agree because she couldn't stop grinning along with him as they glided effortlessly across the urban landscape past Abridge and Chigwell and onward into London.

'Are we going to stop off anywhere?' She asked once they had made it further into the City and were being held back by the volume of traffic.

'To eat you mean? There's some great places to go in Hampstead!'

'No!' Becky dissented, 'well yes, that'll be nice actually, but I meant stop at places your Frank wants you to go to?'

'Not *literally* going to stop at any of those places.' Will answered once he'd eased the car into a stationary position at an awkward junction where the motorway approached the A406.

Becky threw him a quizzical look.

'What's the point then?' She asked.

'I don't know.' Will said absentmindedly as he gave the question some thought. 'Just wasn't planning to that's all.'

'What did Frank say?'

'Only that I should go to these places.'

Will shifted quickly through the gears relishing the burst of the engine as they moved on again.

'You're just being an idiot again aren't you?' Becky said angrily. 'He'd hardly expect you to do a drive-by would he? He probably meant you should stop off and take time to reflect and stuff.'

'Fine.' Will said sullenly. 'But fuck knows where? ...I know he wanted me to go to my old house but what am I supposed to do when we get there? Sit and stare through the windows? That's gonna go down well with the people who live there now innit?'

'But what about where your brother was run over?' Becky suggested.

Will turned to her with a look of pure consternation.

'It's the fucking A1 Becks!' He barked. 'And it was right before you got to a busy roundabout!'

'But shouldn't you at least look at the place for a while?'

'How long's a while? I wouldn't know the exact spot anyway so what's the point?'

Surely you know what the point is? How many times for heaven's sake?' Becky groaned. 'You're supposed to try and feel how you felt when it happened and it hardly matters if you don't know the exact spot does it Will? Just stand on the roundabout and try to soak it up.'

'Okay... if that's what you want I'll do exactly that but all I did was see my brother dead in the road and then I ran away as hard and as fast as I could!'

Becky looked at her husband woefully.

'You've never told me that before,' she said, 'and you're getting upset now aren't you? But that's good though isn't it? That's what's meant to happen.'

'Please Becks,' Will answered, his voice becoming fragmented, 'I know you're only trying to help and I love you for it, but I got enough of that shit off of Frank and I don't need more of it now.'

It was quiet then for a spell as Will concentrated on navigating the car onto the North Circular.

When the lanes were clear and he could relax he gave his wife a fleeting glance out of the corner of his eye. She was watching the road with that stern look she had when she was upset.

'Oh, Becks darling.' He sighed, which was enough to start her sobbing.

'Darling,' he said again, 'I'm *so* sorry, please don't cry… I'll stop everywhere. Let me take you somewhere nice to eat and then we'll go on and I'll stop *everywhere*.'

****

They found a place to eat on the Finchley Road or rather Becky did.

'Look Al Fresco!' She shouted, pointing at the restaurant as they passed, but by the time they'd found a suitable place to park all of the outside tables had been taken.

Only a Pizzeria Will noted with disappointment.

'I'll take you somewhere really nice in Hampstead Village later.' He said looking enviously at the people enjoying lunch in the open air.

'That's if I can ever manage to eat anything ever again.' Becky groaned. 'I'm stuffed.'

'Yeah me too.' Will had to agree.

'So anyway,' Becky said as she pushed away her plate, 'have you made a list of the places we're going to go to?'

'There's Parliament Hill.' Will said. 'We used to fly our kites up there sometimes, although god knows where I'll park.'

'Park a bit away from it.' She suggested. 'I don't mind walking.'

'I know you don't sweetheart.'

'Good, that's one,' she said enthusiastically, 'where else?'

'Well,' he said sedately as he gave the logistics some thought, 'after Parliament Hill we can go further up and then along; there are these really wide paths that have only got that way because people have been treading that route for hundreds of years, thousands maybe, don't know… they take you to these huge open spaces and it's really hard to believe, even when you're a little kid, that somehow you're still in London. There's this flat area, relatively flat anyway, that's covered in tall grass and wild bushes, me and Matt used to play war up there, just the two of us, no one else about. He used to scare the shit out of me, Matt did, crawling away with his gun and I'd be left alone surrounded by all of this tall grass and there'd be these enormous crows jumping around, always screeching and attacking each other. We were a lot more scared of them than they were of us the black bastards, if that's not too racist... so I'd be cowering down with my little gun and Matt would come back and ambush me and shoot me dead or jump me from behind and cut my throat with a lolly stick. I've had many a throat cut up there.' Will reflected with a smile.

'So, it'll be worthwhile reliving those memories wont it?' Becky suggested.

'God yeah,' he sighed, 'I always get nostalgic about being killed.'

'Idiot.'

'I know.'

'What else then?' She asked once they'd turned down the dessert menu and ordered the bill.

'We'll need to go back down and get the car then I'll drive us right to the top of Hampstead. Right to the top of the world I used to think. There's a roundabout up there with a pond in the middle of it that me and Matt went fishing in once, though I think we really will just have to drive by that one what with all the traffic up there, but then we get to cruise down to Highgate. There's a bridge I need to stop at that overlooks where Matt died.'

Will let out a heavy sigh. 'I might get properly sad there though just to warn you.'

'But how many times have I told you that it's the whole idea?' Becky exhorted.

'Thank you Frank.' He said with disdain.

'Sorry.'

'No, *I'm sorry*.' Will said. 'You're right that is the idea. I'm just a little uptight.'

Becky noticed by the strain in his face that he had suddenly become quite tense.

'I think Frank might get a result at the bridge.' He admitted.

Chapter 41 – Man at White Stone Pond

He stood on the plinth of White Stone Pond looking down at the shallow water, disappointment etched all over his face if anyone were there to notice.

He had expected to find the floor of the pond covered with thick foliage just as his memory had pictured it and he'd hoped to see at least one or two gold fish darting in and out of it yet all he had found was a bland bowl almost completely empty of anything other than fallen leaves and assorted litter that washed against the steps on the far side.

He realised then he should never have tested the facts of memories that were steeped so deep in sentiment.

He had got the traffic right, there was still an awful lot of traffic and of course the pub over the road was still standing. Yet, looking around him nothing could be seen to warm his heart or massage his nostalgia as he'd hoped.

He felt himself shivering slightly now. It was still quite a bright day but the wind had clearly picked up since he'd first arrived and now small waves whispered to the perimeter of the pond. The clouds, what there were of them, weren't moving anywhere in a hurry so it was clearly just an anomaly of being up so high.

James knew he'd need to pee in a minute, a chill always did that to him, but where could he go?

Didn't really want to use the pub loo as he always felt obliged to buy a drink if he were spotted by the bar staff and he just couldn't risk the temptation.

The only other choice was to cross the road and find somewhere down the slope. There seemed to be plenty of places he could find privacy down there, a fair amount of trees and a good sprawl of bushes.

It made him doubt his memory to be completely honest. Could there really have been a fairground down there? Given the terrain it hardly seemed possible; barely a level patch of ground to put a coconut shy on let alone the necessary space needed to accommodate the large automated attractions.

Of course, they had found the space somehow. James was aware that his memory may have failed to some degree but his imagination had never been remotely so fanciful.

There had been a 'Whip' somewhere that he and Veronica had ridden on and even a 'Big Wheel' which thankfully she hadn't been so keen to try and a few other examples of crude engineering creaking and straining with age; a Mexican hat he fancied and perhaps a Hearts and Diamonds. But mainly there were stalls as he remembered it, reaching right up from the scraggy bit of field at the bottom to the narrow steps to which he had just now crossed.

James couldn't remember where the goldfish stall had been but had to assume it would have been somewhere near the bottom to afford Veronica the time to come up with the daft scheme of setting each of the little blighters free.

She had actually wanted to go back down to try and win every fish left on the stall once they'd released the two they'd won into the pond.

The idea still made James chuckle now. It would have been a nice thing to do of course, the poor things were kept so badly in those little plastic bags, half of them looking like they were on the verge of death, floating a little lopsided near the surface with nowhere to swim to, but he'd had to break it to her that they'd already spent the best part of a quid winning the two they'd just set free and neither he nor she seemed to have much of a knack with the darts, although, if James recalled correctly, on more than one attempt they had struck the playing cards firmly enough but the dart had popped back out; A sly combination of hard wood frames and horribly blunt darts.

Yes, he remembered now, that was what had made her see reason.

James recollected feeling inside his trouser pocket and rustling the last few pound notes he had between his fingers and wanting to spend it all in a pub, which is exactly what they did in the end.

Crossing over to the Jack Straw's Castle pub, which for some forgotten reason they'd decided to forego, they set off down the other side of the hill hand in hand with the evening sun dazzling them both as it pierced through the lush green branches of the trees.

They had swung their arms back and forth with such velocity that at one point they had both lost their balance momentarily and poor Veronica had nearly slipped into the busy road. Not something that should have been the cause of much merriment but the pair of them were just hysterical with laughter.

They must have looked completely hair brained to the passing motorists but had they cared? No... not a jot.

They were each he was quite sure, so deliriously happy then. James sauntered down the path and found a suitable place to relieve himself and to his surprise he was still shivering even though he had found a well sheltered spot. Perhaps he thought, it was his body's reaction to what his mind had become resolute upon.

He made his way back up the slope and along to the crossing which would take him over to the bus stop to begin his final journey.

He had rather intended to retrace their journey which they had made all those years before and take a walk down the hill to the pub where he and Veronica had finally declared their love for one another on such a wonderful day, but now decided it was better to leave that final memory intact.

Would the pub have still been there? He wondered, and even if it were, the forecourt might be empty even on a day such as today and how sad if all the tables and sun umbrellas had already been packed away for winter. So yes, in reality the decision had made itself.

Now as he stood hard against the bus shelter's advertising board he tried to console himself by softly singing the words of the song that had made their pub so renowned.

'Come, come, come and make eyes at me'
'Down at the Old Bull and Bush'
'Come, come, drink some Port wine with me'
'Down at the Old Bull and Bush'

It didn't take very long, or perhaps it simply didn't seem very long, for the bus to arrive.

Chapter 42 – The bridge

The bus took James through the awkward gap where the Spaniards Inn jutted out across the road having claimed the right when the road had merely been a bridle path many hundreds of years before.

The road was busy now and ran all the way across to Highgate. It was tree lined and there were so many splendid shades of green in that view for him to enjoy as he looked through the grimy window.

When the bus arrived at Highgate Village, James looked around with fondness at the quaint little shops and bistros, gentrified long before the phrase had even been coined.

The affluence of the area confirmed by the Porsches and Mercedes driven by handsome young men or the more mature lady dressed elegantly with sunglasses perched upon the face or swept back leisurely above the forehead.

The feeling of wellbeing he had always felt just being among these people at this place had deserted him now, hardly surprising given the circumstances of this particular visit.

The bus swung right to begin the long stretch downward toward the darker recesses of north London, the deprived crime ridden places which Veronica had once targeted in her grand plan to educate the underprivileged.

He still remembered some of her rhetoric even after all of this time such was her passion. She wanted them all to compete for the better things life could offer, to install ambition, broaden horizons, give them life choices. Regardless of results, he couldn't help but admire her for at least trying.

While he sat contemplating all of this, his stop was suddenly upon him and he had to clamber to press the bell to request the bus to stop. He was very fortunate the driver had deemed to grind the vehicle to a screeching halt at such short notice or he would have been sailing all the way down the hill to Archway station.

Would he have had the compunction to walk all the way back up he wondered?

It only took a moment's consideration and the answer was yes, he would have.

He was here now and this was what he had set out to do come hell or high water. There was absolutely no going back and all he had to do was find a sturdy branch or perhaps a loose piece of fence and he'd be all set.

****

A short while later the Aston Martin was stopped by yet another set of traffic lights and Will could see that just a little further over the brow of the hill there were even more lights to look forward to.

'We're coming up to that pond I was telling you about Becks and by the looks of things we're going to spend more time there than we did at the other two places put together judging by the traffic.'

'It doesn't matter.' She said. 'Don't be grumpy.'

When they'd eventually crawled to the next set they were stopped again on red.

'Look there it is.' Will said pointing onward to the pond.

'Oh my god, it really is a *pond* isn't it?' Becky said in surprise.

'What do you mean?' He asked.

'I just thought it would be much bigger... I mean how can you fish in there? Is it even deep enough?'

Will laughed.

'It's not a proper place for fishing,' he explained, 'we only ever saw two little goldfish in there and Matt and me fished for them with a kid's fishing net like you can get out of Woolworth's.'

'Oh!' she snorted in return, 'I thought they'd be men camped around it in tents with their big fishing rods.'

'Nada.' Will said smiling.

'Did you catch them... the goldfish?'

'One we did.' Will said as they drove off sweeping past the pond and down the Spaniard Inn Road.

'You see this old pub we're coming up to Becks? They reckon Dick Turpin used to stay there and hold up the coaches when they passed.'

Becky gave the slightest nod of her head to feign interest.

252

'Well I hope you'll be a lot more impressed if I can get this thing through the little gap there without getting it smashed up by the oncoming traffic.' He said to tease her.

'You dare!' She retorted. 'We'll have to move into mum's.'
They passed through Highgate and down the hill following the same path trailed by James barely ten minutes earlier.

Will indicated left and entered Hornsey Lane toward the bridge. Becky suddenly noticed how solemn he'd become.

'You okay?' She asked.
'Yeah,' he answered cheerlessly, 'I'm just thinking about where to park.'

'Oh good,' she said, 'you had me worried.'
'I'm fine sweetheart.' He said without any conviction.

They passed a row of houses and the boys' college and were soon at the mouth of the bridge.

'Have a look left at the view.' Will urged her, while keeping his own eyes firmly on the road ahead.

Becky turned her head and felt the fresh sweep of thermal air on her face.

'Oh look! there's someone up there Will!' She suddenly shrieked.

'That's probably just that weird gargoyle thing in the middle.' Will suggested, having quickly recovered from the start she'd given him.

'No, I'm telling you! There's someone right up on the edge hanging over!'
Will glanced quickly into the rear-view mirror but couldn't see anything.

'You sure?' He asked.
'Yes, *definitely!*'

At a point in the road just past the bridge the car swerved and mounted the kerb with a heavy crunch then screeched to an abrupt halt.

'Shit! What are you *doing!*' Becky screamed.

'That's a jumper.' Will said calmly as he unfastened his seatbelt and swung the door open in one smooth movement before leaping out of the car.

'Where are you going!' Becky berated.

'I'm gonna try and stop whoever it is!' Will shouted behind him, as he walked determinedly toward the bridge.

He glanced at the view for the first time since he was a child, the whole of the City before him, the huge Natwest Tower, The Stock Exchange by its side, St Paul's Cathedral and somewhere to one side the odd shape of The Post Office Tower.

Looking up and along the bridge itself he came across the stone column at its centre and at the large cast iron lamp rising skyward wrapped as it was by iron dolphins that he only remembered vaguely as being gargoyles.

Becks had been right! James could see a figure clinging precariously with both hands to the lamplight's pole.

The man, it was clearly a man, had half of his backside on the flat stone and had stretched a leg out which he'd wedged between the spikes at the top of the cast iron fencing.

To Will's untrained mind he looked more intent on saving himself than flinging himself off.

When Will had got close he had to cover his face with a forearm to shield his eyes from the sun to get a proper look at him and hopefully make some eye contact.

'You alright mate!' He asked, then cursed himself immediately for beginning with such a ludicrous question.

'Please just go away.' James pleaded shakily, without properly bothering to see who he was talking to.

'I can't,' Will reasoned, 'I've got to get you down.'

'*Look,* I know you mean well and it's very kind of you but *please*... I don't want your help.'

'Understood.' Will said calmly as he stepped a little further forward toward the fence grill.

James began visibly trembling now and was feeling so much worse than he was before this character involved himself and he could feel his grip on the lamppost begin to weaken.

'Fuck off now will you!' He shouted hoping to sound assertive. 'I'm not ready yet!'

'If I walk away you'll come down?' Will asked hopefully.

But it wasn't what James meant. He just needed a little more time for reflection and to find the final spurt of courage he needed to jump. He had been okay until then, relatively speaking, sitting still as he was. No one had seemed to notice him until this idiot came along, but now the traffic had slowed to a crawl as everyone became a fucking spectator. Worse still there was someone else coming to aid him.

Becky stood beside her husband and brushed his sleeve with her hand as a gesture of support.

'Will you come down if I walk away?' Will asked again. 'Or I can stay and help you down.' He said, as he took a more detailed look at the railings.

'How the hell did you get up there anyway?'

'I can assure you it wasn't easy.' James snapped indignantly. 'I had to jam several pieces of wood through the grates at intervals to make steps... no point you even trying now, I felt one of them snap as I lifted my foot from it and anyway I could quite easily dislodge you if you came near.'

Will inspected the grill and sure enough noticed the pieces of wood.

'Trust me,' he said ardently, 'I won't be getting up there, I don't like heights as it is. Just standing here is bad enough.'

'Then don't bloody stand there!' James shouted down angrily turning his back completely on Will and letting one hand free.

'Wow! Wait! *Please wait!*' Will cried desperately. 'Just listen for a minute... before the police come, because they're gonna come aren't they?'

'Why on earth aren't they here already?' Becky whispered.

'Before they come,' Will said, ignoring her, 'I just want to tell you something about myself... well, about my brother really, you see he died on that road down there, just on the turn of the bend at the bottom and he was only eleven. It very nearly ruined the whole of my life.'

Becky took Will's hand and gave it a squeeze.

'Haven't you got a family mate? Isn't there someone's life you're gonna ruin?' He asked.

James turned back around with menacing eyes looking very much like he had something to say but nothing was forthcoming.

'My brother didn't have the choice like you've got.' Will continued vehemently, 'He was run over you see, no one's fault really but you never get over it however much you try to stop thinking about it, it's always there.'

James began whimpering in desperation, his face shrivelled and twisted. 'Fuck off.' He uttered inaudibly.

'I'm going to go and find a phone box to call nine, nine, nine in case no one else has.' Becky whispered again, releasing Will's hand and walking away at a pace.

'So, have you got a family mate?' Will began to probe.
James rolled his eyes skywards but nodded.

'And you don't care how much doing this is gonna hurt them?'
'They won't care!' James suddenly blurted out.

'Is that what you think? I mean who are these people who wouldn't be bothered if you died?' They're not your *close* family are they?'

'They're my children!' James conceded.
'Okay.' Will said, immediately trying to find some leverage. 'They're teenagers I'm guessing? Not the best lot to communicate with are they? If you're properly down and you've even told them you're down they probably didn't take you seriously, might not even have listened, it's a lot...'

'They're not teenagers they're little boys!'
'Oh,' Will said looking up at the older man disconcertedly.

'Then why wouldn't they care if their dad dies? What makes you think they know how much they need you?'

'I've nothing they need that I can give them... I'm not allowed to *see* them, I have no money to *support* them... and there are other things... things that I just can't discuss.'

Will was saddened by those remarks, saddened for every little child who would grow up strange, complicated and yet painfully dull through the actions of their mums and their dads.

It seemed incredibly unfair when the complications that would shape their lives weren't even theirs to understand. The loneliness that would be thrust upon them by a parent too engrossed in the misery or failures of their own existence. Surely, they could at least strive for redemption through the lives of their children?

He looked around him to make sure Becks hadn't returned and then he took a moment just to check the sudden surge of emotion that had hit him as he began to consider the words he was about to say.

He stepped a little closer to the fencing as if to talk to James in confidence although he still needed to raise his voice to be heard.

'I'm going to tell you something else that I haven't even managed to tell my wife yet.' He began. 'I even had a shrink and I couldn't tell him because I knew if I said it aloud it would be real and I didn't... I don't want it to be real. Can you understand that?'

James nodded ever so slightly.

'Well then... you see, if you do what you're about to do your kids are gonna need a shrink too. My dad you see... after my brother died, he couldn't handle it... and when I needed a dad more than ever and when my poor old mum needed a husband he came up here and he threw himself off this fucking bridge!'

Will suddenly found himself crying, effortlessly, tears running down his face and rich effluence from his nose and he could have actually howled then and welcomed such a mournful release but he held onto his breathing and fought for control of his voice as he had more he needed to say.

'I can't ever forgive him mate.' He spluttered. 'I was just a little boy and my poor old mum might just as well have died herself after he did that but she didn't. She carried on for me, she didn't even burden me with it and she carried on... you know you shouldn't do it! It's not fair mate... you shouldn't do it!'

Will had become so absorbed in sorrow that he didn't notice James move or see him swing a leg around and make the leap.

A woman screamed and Will, suddenly alert, looked around instinctively at the pedestrian queue of traffic to find her.

One man had clearly flinched at something and another had that sullen look of disappointment on his face.

Could it only have been Will who missed the thud as James descended with knees grasped onto the pavement almost beside him.

Will had merely followed the eyes of the onlookers who in unison were watching James sit up and now Will in shock had bolted the short distance to his aid and had an arm under one of James's armpits and the second wrapped around James's arm to pull him upright to a standing position.

James had clearly hurt himself judging by the pained expression on his face but he hadn't uttered a word.

'Take your time.' Will suggested as he carefully brought James upright before gently releasing him from his grasp.

'Thank you.' Will said sincerely. 'You should be proud of yourself for fighting the urge you must have had... you know that?'

James didn't answer and he didn't even look at Will to acknowledge him, he simply stood there with his head bowed and his eyes fixed firmly on the pavement before him.

Becky had found a phone box on the corner and had made her call to the emergency services before returning.

She moved sedately by her husband's side.

'So pleased he's down.' She whispered, as she inspected the strange man from behind Will's shoulder.

'They're coming.' She whispered again, referring to the emergency services, then as Will turned to her she noticed his blotchy face.

'Shit are you okay?' She asked. 'Have you been crying?'

'Look it doesn't matter.' Will said quickly before brushing his arm across his face to wipe away the tears. 'But what are we going to do now?' He asked.

'We'll just have to keep him calm and make sure he doesn't get away.' Becky suggested.

'No!' Will growled and clutched his head in frustration.

'We can't just let the police or the ambulance or whoever it is who's coming just cart him off... he'll be back to square one Becks.'

'What are you talking about then?' She asked.

'I don't know yet.'

'And have you been crying?'

'Yeah I have, but I'll tell you about that later... I've got a lot to tell you later sweetheart, but look, I don't want them to take him.'

'Oh for God sakes Will what is it now!' She complained venomously.

'Look, I'm sorry, I'm really, really sorry, but I want to help him properly. When I explain everything you'll understand sweetheart... It'll be good therapy for me.'

'But *how* can we help him Will?'

'We can help him escape, we can give him some money for a new start.'

'But we're boracic ourselves now darling.' Becky reminded him.

'We'll find some money, something'll come up, it always does.'

'*Really?*' Becky answered in a cynical tone.

'I bloody hope so.' Will said.

'But how can we even get him away from here?'

'He'll just have to squeeze into the back.'

'Of *that* car?' Becky wondered in disbelief.

'Yes.'

'You're not bloody kidding he'll have to squeeze in!'

'It's doable.' Will argued sincerely.

Becky stood in silence, a quizzical look on her face as she considered the logistics being suggested then suddenly they could both hear sirens.

She looked at Will and frowned.

'Go on then you idiot.' She sighed. 'Those must be for him.'

Will ran to her and hugged her, quickly lifting her into the air and around before moving onto James who had been standing perfectly still all of that time, head still bowed.

'What's your name mate?' He asked hurriedly.

'James.' Was the very sombre response.

'Hello James.' Will said thrusting out his hand and shaking the quivering appendage that had moved tentatively toward him.

'I'm Will and that amazing lady over there is my wife Rebecca... so tell me James, do you like fast cars?'

Printed in Great Britain
by Amazon